T0227788

CULTURE, HEALTH AND DISEASE

TAVISTOCK

The International Behavioural and Social Sciences Library

HEALTH & SOCIETY
In 12 Volumes

CULTURE, HEALTH AND DISEASE

Social and Cultural Influences on Health Programmes in Developing Countries

MARGARET READ

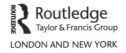

Routledge
Taylor & Francis Group

LONDON AND NEW YORK

First published in 1966 by
Tavistock Publications Limited

Published in 2001 by
Routledge
2 Park Square, Milton Park, Abingdon, Oxfordshire OX14 4RN
711 Third Avenue, New York, NY 10017

First issued in paperback 2014

Routledge is an imprint of the Taylor and Francis Group, an informa business

British Library Cataloguing in Publication Data
A CIP catalogue record for this book
is available from the British Library

Culture, Health and Disease
ISBN 0-415-26430-8
Health & Society: 12 Volumes
ISBN 0-415-26509-6
The International Behavioural and Social Sciences Library
112 Volumes
ISBN 0-415-25670-4

ISBN 13: 978-1-138-88138-9 (pbk)
ISBN 13: 978-0-415-26430-3 (hbk)

MARGARET READ

Culture, Health, and Disease

SOCIAL AND CULTURAL INFLUENCES
ON HEALTH PROGRAMMES
IN DEVELOPING COUNTRIES

TAVISTOCK PUBLICATIONS
LONDON SYDNEY TORONTO WELLINGTON

First published in 1966
by Tavistock Publications Limited
2 Park Square, Milton Park, Abingdon, Oxon, OX14 4RN
in 10 pt Plantin, 2 pt leaded
by Richard Clay (The Chaucer Press) Ltd
Bungay, Suffolk
© Margaret Read, 1966

Contents

Contents

Contents

Preface

Since the publication of 'Social and cultural backgrounds for planning public health programmes in Africa' (Read, 1957), public health administrators, and medical and nursing personnel responsible for training, have asked the writer for a book describing the social anthropologist's interpretation of the varying reactions of different groups of people to public health programmes. They felt that such a book would provide at least a partial explanation of some of the problems they encountered in their work. At a conference of the International Union for Health Education in Philadelphia in July 1962, after a key address by the writer on 'Man in his social environment' (Read, 1962), these requests were renewed.

With the help of a grant from the Milbank Memorial Fund the book was planned, and illustrative material was collected from a number of sources. These sources include the writer's personal experience and field research in several tropical countries; contacts with health workers and social scientists; discussions with WHO personnel in Geneva and elsewhere; and published papers and books which, together with some unpublished material, are listed in the references. The scope of the book is limited to problems of health and disease in rural areas of developing countries, for the most part in tropical regions. Illustrative material includes actual health situations and the results of medical and social science research into popular response to programmes.

A note is perhaps necessary about the selection of material. Primarily it was selected to show cooperation in research by health personnel and social scientists, and the application of this research to implementing specific health programmes and to training health personnel. If some studies have been drawn on heavily it is because this cooperation was effectively demonstrated in the published material. Medical and other teachers, who might reject this material because it appears not to apply to them directly, could use it to stimulate similar studies in their own areas, as well as to illustrate techniques of study and analysis of current problems.

Acknowledgements

Thanks are due to the following individuals and institutions for permission to quote material from the sources listed below:

J. Adair, International Universities Press, Inc., and the New York Academy of Medicine in respect of 'Physicians, medicine men and their Navaho patients' in *Man's image in medicine and anthropology* edited by I. Galdston; J. Adair, K. Deuschle, W. McDermott, and the American Academy of Political and Social Science in respect of 'Patterns of health and disease among the Navahos'; H. Ammar and Routledge & Kegan Paul Ltd in respect of *Growing up in an Egyptian village*; H. Ammar and the Arab States Fundamental Education Centre in respect of 'The sociological approach to problems of community development'; A. Burgess and the American Public Health Association in respect of 'Nutrition education in public health programmes: what have we learned?'; S. C. Dube and Routledge & Kegan Paul Ltd in respect of *Indian village*; M. J. Field and Faber & Faber Ltd in respect of *Search for security*; G. M. Foster and the Social Science Research Council in respect of 'Problems in intercultural health programmes'; L. P. Gerlach and the Minnesota Academy of Science in respect of 'Economy and protein malnutrition among the Digo'; J. J. Groen, D. Ben-Ishay, B. I. Ben-Assa, and the Editor of *Voeding* in respect of 'Clinical and biochemical osteomalacia among the Bedouin of the Negev desert'; R. S. Khare and the Editor of *Human Organization* in respect of 'Folk medicine in a North Indian village'; T. A. Lambo and Ibadan University Press in respect of 'African traditional beliefs, concepts of health and medical practice'; M. L. Lantis and Oregon State University in respect of 'American Arctic populations: their survival problem'; J. B. Loudon and the Central Council of Health Education in respect of 'Social structure and health concepts among the Zulu'; F. Maxwell Lyons and the Editor of *The Practitioner* in respect of 'Trachoma'; W. McDermott, K. Deuschle, J. Adair, H. Fulmer, B. Loughlin, and the Editor of *Science* in respect of 'Introducing modern medicine in a Navaho community (Copyright 1960 by the American Association for the

Acknowledgements

Advancement of Science); J. C. Messenger and The University of Chicago Press in respect of 'Religious acculturation among the Anang-Ibibio' in *Continuity and change in African cultures* edited by W. Bascom and M. J. Herskovits; M. E. Opler and the Editor of *Human Organization* in respect of 'The cultural definition of illness in village India'; Oxford University Press in respect of *The Ngoni of Nyasaland* by Margaret Read (published under the auspices of the International African Institute); D. R. Price-Williams and the Editor of the *International Journal of Health Education* in respect of 'New attitudes emerge from old' ('The changing ideas of health and disease among the Tiv of Central Nigeria'); L. Saunders and the American Public Health Association, Western Regional Office, in respect of 'The contributions and limitations of behavioral sciences in public health' in *The behavioral sciences and public health*; N. L. Solien, H. S. Scrimshaw, and the Editor of the *Journal of Tropical Pediatrics* in respect of 'Public health significance of child feeding practices observed in a Guatemalan village'; F. V. Tentori and the Editor of the *International Journal of Health Education* in respect of 'Their needs and knowledge'; B. B. Waddy and the Royal Society of Tropical Medicine and Hygiene in respect of 'The present state of public health in the African Soudan'; M. Wilson and Oxford University Press in respect of *Rituals of kinship among the Nyakyusa* (published under the auspices of the International African Institute); World Health Organization, Regional Office for Africa, in respect of 'Social and cultural backgrounds for planning public health programmes in Africa' by Margaret Read.

Introduction

In one developing country after another governments are planning the extension of all kinds of services to rural areas which were formerly neglected. Building roads, establishing rural health centres, introducing better seeds and fertilizers, opening schools, providing water supplies, setting up loud-speaker radios – these are some of the many new government activities and rural services intended to raise the level of living. The local health worker, doctor, nurse, or sanitary engineer thus becomes one of several innovators introducing socio-economic changes, and is so regarded by the people. Village people, who have their own image of government, may be afraid of officials and of the punishment that may follow non-compliance with regulations. They may also believe, on the basis of past experience, that governments are indifferent to the sufferings of people living in remote areas, and this may cause them to regard the intentions of these new officials with suspicion.

EFFECTS OF RURAL ISOLATION

The tide of socio-economic change, however, has not yet reached everywhere. All over the tropical areas are communities whose isolation has cut them off from new developments. Thus people may live in the rice lands of South-East Asia, where villages can be reached only by walking on the tops of bunds between the rice fields; they may live in a clearing in an African forest penetrated only by red laterite footpaths; they may live in the savannah lands on the edge of deserts where hardly distinguishable sandy tracks stretch away into the distance. Whatever their geographical environment, these villages 'beyond the end of the road' have some common characteristics that profoundly affect the wellbeing and ill health of the people, and their response to the health services that are able to reach them.

In the first place, their physical isolation from main roads, motor traffic, and large centres of population forces them to practise a largely subsistence economy; to regulate their own internal affairs; and to rely on mutual help in cases of sickness.

This self-reliance is based on their ecological adjustment to their environment and their familiarity with the insecurities of their surroundings. They have learned to face periods of drought, occasional flooding, erosion of their soil, attacks on their food crops from baboons, birds, locusts, and other invaders. In this environment where they have achieved a 'delicate balance' they have had to satisfy their basic needs for food, water, fuel, and remedies to cure illnesses. They have long been acquainted with chronic or seasonal hunger, with a high child death-rate related to malnutrition, and with chronic ill health from infestations and the after-effects of diseases such as malaria, cholera, and pneumonia.

Health workers trained on scientific medical lines perceive immediately the magnitude of the need for health services in these rural tropical areas. Whether they are familiar or unfamiliar with the prevailing health problems, they are often unaware of the nature of the 'delicate balance' achieved by local populations. When health workers inject their modern remedies for ill health in a piecemeal fashion, without taking into account the complex of activities that make up the life of a rural community, they may be baffled by the apparent lack of response from the people.

THE ROLE OF THE SOCIAL SCIENCES

Faced with familiar or unfamiliar problems in rural tropical areas, health workers have turned to social scientists for help in understanding people's reactions to health programmes, as the following quotations show:

Dr Lyle Saunders, an American anthropologist with experience of Latin American health problems, writes:

'The historical association and the recent emerging convergence of interest between behavioral science and public health derive from two obvious, but fundamental, aspects of the nature of health and of public health activity:

'1. Social and cultural behaviors are important factors in the etiology, prevalence, and distribution of many diseases. How people live, what they eat, what they believe, what they value, what technology they command, are significant determinants of their individual and collective health.

'2. Public health is a social and cultural activity. Both its practitioners and the human targets of its services are, in their various

xiv

interactions and transactions, fulfilling socially-defined roles in culturally determined ways, and a good deal of their behavior is motivated, oriented and constrained by the social and cultural contexts in which it occurs' (Saunders, 1962).

Dr Hamed Ammar, an Egyptian sociologist, and Director of Training in the Arab States Fundamental Education Centre, refers to the need for research, also to the cultural implications of changes caused by public health programmes:

'Planning health programs involves the study of present resources, the sizing up of the actual conditions and the setting of targets and objectives to be achieved over a given time in the light of a clear social philosophy. Operationally, this implies better use of existing resources, meeting, changing and redirecting present needs, and creating new ones.

'Comprehensive planning requires the preparation of all social forces to be encountered or anticipated. Health programs have to be seen in their perspective as related to economic conditions, educational factors, population problems, family patterns, and material and human resources. All this necessitates continued social research. Sound planning of health programs must be integrated with other social and economic activities. Public health planning must make the fullest use of research both on the national and local levels if it is to strike roots and achieve results. . . . The organization of social research must be considered as an integral part of the public health programs.

'People in countries characterized by a slow rate of change have adopted certain health practices, habits, medicaments and a general view of health along certain traditional lines. What often appears to be the dogged adherence of conservative people to harmful ways is not pure stubbornness – it is just that the new changes advocated do not "make sense" to them . . . There can be no escape from facing and solving the cultural equation of medicine, health, illness and treatment' (Ammar, 1960).

Health workers and social scientists alike recognize that response to health services and programmes in rural areas depends upon deliberate choice by people. Making decisions about actions to be taken and weighing one choice against another are familiar procedures in day-to-day rural life. But the new demands by government agencies for cooperation in successive development programmes of one kind and another impose on rural communities and on the individuals in them new and heavy burdens.

Dr Saber, a Sudanese anthropologist, describes the potential confusion of people faced with many changes directed from above, and suggests that the absence of continuity with a people's traditional way of living imposes stresses on the individual and on his society:

'Our developing societies are passing through a crucial transition period in the unavoidable battle caused by the very nature of contemporary life, the complicated functions of the modern state and the determination of the individual to keep up his dignity in today's life.
. . . To these societies the present seems rather alien, for it cannot be considered a continuation of their past history. Indeed, it is a new epoch that seems to have been cut off from the tide of time, with almost no relation to the past' (Saber, 1962, p. 6).

Dr Tentori, a Mexican physician who has served with international agencies, carries the concept of a new and alien epoch opening up for rural communities into a plea for greater understanding of the traditional background of people:

'Generally, when we undertake education for health, we very often forget the economic situation, the interests, the needs, the wishes, the problems, the knowledge of the individual or group concerned. We also forget that our way of thinking, knowledge, our attitudes, are the result of academic training that we acquired at school, from the first grade to University, and . . . we try to communicate our knowledge as if the people concerned had something of our preparation.

'We express the contents of our educational messages, using the knowledge that we ourselves have, which is very different and sometimes even opposite to that of the people. In other instances, we act as if the persons concerned had no knowledge, and we forget then that they have accumulated through the years a series of experiences that represent a world of knowledge.

'While our training as health specialists has been partly systematic, the people have acquired their whole knowledge in situations of life, and not in books or conferences' (Tentori, 1962).

PLAN OF THE BOOK

This is the point at which the main themes of the book are taken up.

Part I covers the essential background for understanding people's reactions to modern health programmes. The hazards to health inherent in an exacting and often hostile tropical environment are related to people's own attempts to deal with sickness and to preserve a measure of health. These practices are presented here as a 'system of traditional care' for sick people, incorporating the concept of folk medicine and the methods of divination and healing, together with the relation of 'traditional practitioners' to modern medical personnel.

In Parts II and III some of the methods and findings of social scientists who have studied these traditional systems are explained. The recognition of the dual process of social change and social continuity and its relation to the ambivalence of people's response to health programmes is emphasized as an essential in the training of health personnel for work in rural areas.

PART I

Traditional systems of care in sickness

CHAPTER I

Survival studies and health hazards

TECHNIQUES FOR SURVIVAL IN A HARSH ENVIRONMENT

Around the beginning of this century, some of the early anthropologists studied the aborigines in Central Australia, and discovered a relationship between their social organization, their food quest, and their religious ritual. These small aboriginal bands wrested a living from an unpropitious environment through hunting and through collecting grubs and roots. They built up what they regarded as a measure of security through rituals which linked each band to an area and to the possible food to be found there, and ensured continuity and preservation through a system of seasonal ceremonies and taboos. The food quest was of such vital importance to the aboriginal population that all their life was organized around it; and measures of severe social discipline were enforced in the small communities to ensure that no one individual exploited the scarce resources so as to deprive his fellows of the necessary food for keeping alive.

Archaeological evidence has shown that the Eskimo in his Arctic habitat has survived for more than 2,000 years with a material culture and manner of living which were common to many small groups. The similarity of their language and non-material culture suggests that these groups may have been in touch with each other from time to time, and able to move from one locality to another, as the quest for food demanded.

Before western nations pushed into the Arctic and made certain demands upon the local people and their environment, the Eskimo found his food, clothing, shelter, light, fuel, and medicines in that environment. In a paper on survival problems of American Arctic populations Dr Margaret Lantis lists the techniques which were used by the Eskimo to assure a food supply. Besides moving in a seasonal pattern within a defined area, the Eskimo had

'a remarkable range of techniques for storing food: for example, dried, frozen, kept frozen or unfrozen in containers made of whole

3

sealskin, animal stomach or other pouch, in stone, wood or pottery vessel . . . or in a pit in the ground. Food was placed on racks, in wooden storehouses, in ice caves, or in the house itself. Besides mammals, the birds and their eggs, fish and their eggs, greens, roots and berries, shell fish, octopus (in the Aleutians), and crustaceans were eaten if their presence was known; and there were customary methods of storing most of them . . . Recognizing food was one of the adaptive skills of a frontier people' (Lantis, 1957, p. 125).

Studies of health conditions among the Somali in the arid region of north-east Africa bring out the rigours of a nomadic life for people dependent on their herds and the need to find pasture and water for them. The perpetual search for water governs their migrations, regulated by those watering places where there is a permanent supply, and now by the additional cisterns or tanks that are being built, to which water is carried in trucks. Food for humans is always short, though there is a strong belief that milk, the chief element in their diet, is the only food that can sustain life by itself. Among the women there is a high fertility rate, but there is also a high rate of infant mortality. In a report on a study of heart disease among Somali tribesmen (WHO, 1963a), doctors in the capital of Somalia tried to establish a relationship between the diet, consisting almost entirely of camel's milk, and the extreme rarity of atherosclerotic conditions. They concluded that, in spite of the simplicity and monotony of the diet, physical development is good and shows a remarkable power of resistance to hard and demanding living conditions. They also considered that the people live in accordance with century-old custom, and are emotionally balanced and free from nervous tension because their way of living is closely adapted to the surrounding conditions, into which they were born and in which they will remain all their lives.

There are certain conclusions to be drawn from this brief look at survival in harsh and isolated environments. First, the people learned to adjust their forms of livelihood to the limitations of their surroundings, in which their basic needs for food, shelter, and care for their health had to be met; second, the people were organized in relatively small groups, and so preserved their mobility in search of food and water; third, they accepted the rigours of their life and believed in the value of establishing harmony with their environment through rituals and ceremonies.

SOME TYPICAL ENVIRONMENTAL HAZARDS

Most tropical areas illustrate the hazards to people's health arising from the contamination or shortage of water; from the scarcity or imbalance of food supplies; and from infections and infestations arising from the environment.

Water shortage

In the French-speaking Soudan the outstanding need is for an international project to ensure

'improved rural water supplies in the campaign against contact diseases, particularly yaws, endemic syphilis and leprosy. It may seem a mere flight of fancy to envisage a copious (not necessarily purified) water supply in every village of the Soudan. But no other public health project can compare with this in value. The water exists, in rivers, swamps and underground: all that is needed is the money and the engineers to carry it to human settlements' (Waddy, 1962, p. 108).

Food shortage

In rural areas poorer families always have a difficult choice in deciding how to spend their small amount of cash. In a South India nutrition survey (Someswara Rao *et al.*, 1959) 79 per cent of the rural families had incomes of Rs 50 and under per month. Eighty-two per cent of these families had cases of marasmus or protein-calorie deficiency conditions in their children. Their habitual diet of cooked cereals, eaten once or at most twice daily, with vegetables added sometimes only twice a week, could have been augmented by milk from their own cow or buffalo. But 90 per cent of the milk produced in these households was sold for cash needed for essential purchases.

Environmental diseases

A constant challenge to human health in the tropics comes from the diseases that arise from the biological environment of human settlements. One of the papers at the IUHE conference mentioned in the Preface described the malaria-eradication service in Ethiopia (Zelleke, 1962). Here, the basic reason for the underdevelopment of fertile areas was the existence of malaria, since 60 per cent of the land surface, most

5

of it fertile valleys and plains, was actually or potentially malarious. Three pilot projects with their extensions had resulted in some 500,000 people, as well as new settlers in improved land areas, now living well protected from malaria. In Viet Nam a malaria-eradication team found that the women and children went to live on the rice fields to protect the crops until the harvest was over. An examination of the children showed that those living in the villages where the houses had been sprayed had a spleen rate of 4·7 and a parasite rate of 6; whereas the children living on the fields had comparable rates of 80 and 55. Here, obviously, the malaria-eradication programme would have to include spraying the temporary huts on the rice fields in order to adapt the programme to the necessary migration of the people from the village sites to protect their food supply. The same kind of situation was found to exist in Ceylon, Burma, and Thailand.

In parts of Africa, human sleeping sickness is still an environmental menace, and its control demands perpetual vigilance:

'Human sleeping sickness . . . is a disease of very slow onset. Often there is an interval of two years between infection and the onset of symptoms: during all this period the unwitting sufferer carries trypanosomes in his blood and is infectious to vector tsetse flies. Africans are great travellers, without respect for the frontiers elaborated by nineteenth, and now twentieth, century politics, and sleeping sickness is spread by human carriers. The vector tsetses require a humid microclimate. In the dry zones they exist only in very close proximity to water; since everyone uses the same river crossings and waterholes, man-fly contact is perfect, and an infected traveller can start a chain of epidemics along his route. Even if the treatment, and where to get it, are well known, only a small proportion of sleeping sickness victims find their way to a hospital or treatment centre, and this is therefore a disease that can wipe out entire populations' (Waddy, 1962).

Another environmental disease with an intermediate host – a snail – associated with water is schistosomiasis or bilharziasis. It is recognized as second in importance to malaria as a parasitic disease, and hence is a major public health problem wherever it occurs. It has a high incidence in younger age groups, since children become infected from two years on, and it affects both their physical and mental development. It diminishes the productive power and physical strength of adults and

6

saps resistance to other infections. As an increasing environmental health hazard it is closely connected with opening up more cultivatable land through irrigation, as in Egypt, where the disease has existed in the Nile Valley for centuries:

'With the existing pattern of rural life in Egypt, contact with snail-infested water is not only highly probable but more often than not inevitable. Very early in life, children accompany their mothers to canals for domestic activities. They are fond of playing in shallow water. At school age, rural children take to swimming in canals as a main summer entertainment practice. Later on, rural life practices bring the people to canals for irrigation, fishing, bathing animals, washing, filling jars, washing crops, and for many other domestic and occupational purposes.'[1]

The fly, *Simulium damnosum*, the cause of onchocerciasis or 'river blindness', is another environmental enemy to man:

'The effects of onchocerciasis in a hyperendemic area include high rates of blindness affecting chiefly the adult males in their prime, who should be forming the labour force; also pruritis of such severity as to lead to suicide. . . . There is no doubt that hyperendemic onchocerciasis and its diabolic little vector cause retreat from the river valleys with which it is associated. . . .

'Consider the fate of a placid, fertile river valley in the African savannah, after a primitive agricultural community settles in it. Primitive farming, with its technique of grass-burning, inevitably leads to soil erosion. As soil erosion starts, the run-off of rainwater into the river becomes more precipitate, rocks start to appear, and *Simulium damnosum* starts to breed on a large scale. The combination of soil erosion and the *Simulium* nuisance causes a human retreat from the river, and so the process of creating soil erosion and new *Simulium* breeding grounds is carried further and further up the watershed until the whole valley is depopulated and eroded' (Waddy, 1962, pp. 103–4).

TRADITIONAL RESPONSES TO ILL HEALTH

Hazards to health exist everywhere. Some are man made, as the 'smog' in urban centres. Others arise from biological and physical

[1] Personal communication.

7

environments hitherto unconquered. They range from extremes of heat or cold or lack of water to local infestations and infections which modern science is slowly discovering how to control. In most tropical areas health hazards loom large in the lives of the inhabitants and take a heavy toll in death and disability. The populations of these areas have developed some degree of self-reliance, and have endeavoured to use their empirical knowledge acquired by trial and error to cope with the heavy rates of sickness and death.

To deal with this burden of recurrent sickness, they have built up systems of folk medicine and traditional care for the sick. Health personnel working in these areas sooner or later discover the existence of folk medicine, and observing certain ineffective manifestations of its practice they are inclined to be scornful of its remedies. As a rule it appears to them as a series of odd 'customs', and they are at a loss to relate one 'custom' to another, or to understand the reasoning that motivates certain actions and underlies firmly held beliefs. These beliefs and practices often endure in spite of the availability of modern medical care, which is accepted in many areas where rural people have learned to welcome its successful curative services.

Social scientists have studied ways of analysing these traditional systems, so that they can be understood not as a collection of customs with no coherent meaning, but as complexes of social relationships and cultural patterns of behaviour and thought. There appear to be three basic elements in these systems of traditional aid in sickness:

1. The social structure and social organization of the people, from which arise the nature and degree of the mutual dependence of individuals in sickness and in health, in childhood and in age, and their respect for and dependence on those who are recognized as possessing certain traditional skills as healers.

2. The methods of treatment in sickness and the measures taken to prevent and ward off accidents and illness.

3. The concepts of the natural and the supernatural world, which give people some basis for their beliefs about the onset of sickness, the likelihood of cure, and the preservation of health.

CHAPTER 2

Role of the kin group in illness

As medical care and modern public health programmes reach out in effective and permanent units to the remoter rural areas, the problems of the health personnel who work in these rural units emerge, and appear to be far more complicated than those encountered in urban centres. There, advice and treatment are given in clinics and hospitals to which patients have come voluntarily and where they are, at least physically, under the control of the professional health personnel. The health worker in a rural area becomes aware, perhaps for the first time, of the existence of another 'medical care' system based on ideas about the causes and treatment of disease evolved over long years of experience by the people in terms of their environment, their pattern of living, and their beliefs about human, environmental, and supernatural relationships.

Let us suppose that the health worker is able to visit the villages and people's homes and extend his knowledge at present limited to seeing patients in the setting of the health centre or mobile clinic. Careful observation and some discreet questioning will show that, in a village, when a person is taken ill, he turns to people related to him who live in the same household or in nearby households. These may consult other relations in the village, and in the wider group of kin who live in neighbouring settlements. What is the role of this narrower or wider kin group in relation to the sick person?

The first thing the kinsfolk do is to take notice of the illness, take care of and comfort the sick person, and make him feel that he has support in his suffering. Other members of his kin group may be called in to observe the symptoms, and if these do not yield to the home remedies that are advised, they decide to call a 'specialist' from among the traditional practitioners. Members of the kin group are present at the consultation with the 'specialist', carry out whatever treatment he prescribes, and report back to him about the effects of the treatment. If it is successful they are responsible for paying the 'specialist' whatever the agreed reward might be; and if unsuccessful they will consult him again, and maybe he will advise going to another 'specialist' or to a modern hospital.

Supportive elements

Among the Navaho Indians of the United States:

> 'The individual who is sick does not act on his own. The family is likely to take matters into its own hands once its members know that one of their number is sick. After the diagnostician has indicated the root of the illness he suggests what *sing* should be performed; then the family goes off for a *singer* who knows the required ceremony, and they arrange with him what the fee for the *sing* shall be. No ceremonies are performed free of charge – a payment is essential for the efficacy of treatment.
>
> 'Furthermore the family is all present while the *sing* is in progress; it may last from one to nine nights, depending on the nature of the illness for which the *sing* is given, the economic position of the family, and other factors. Relatives and friends come to the ceremony and take part in the chants and prayers directed by the medicine man and his assistant. By association they too receive positive benefits from the cure, and in turn the presence of the family and friends is assuring to the patient who feels they are all working to restore his health' (Adair, 1963).

Navaho decisions about what actions to take are made as a rule by the matrilineal relatives, that is by the wife's father and mother if they are living, who may talk it over with the man's family also, since all of them help to prepare for the *sing*. The man may have already been to the hospital and not responded to treatment there, and so the family tries the hand trembler or 'diagnostician' to find out if anything further will help.

Among the Tiv in Central Nigeria:

> 'In relation to health and sickness the indigenous picture was that of diviners, herbalists and men that performed special rituals. Sickness is generically known by the term *akombo*. Basically *akombo* are non-human forces that can be manipulated by people. They are also magical emblems, symbolised by a pot or stick, or plant, and so on. . . .

Role of the kin group in illness

As regards illness, *akombo* stands for the symptoms of a disease, and can therefore be differentiated into various syndromes designated by a separate name. If a person falls ill, particularly if it is persistent or very serious, it is assumed that an *akombo* has "caught" him. He consults a diviner who advises him what to do. This means calling together either his father's kin, or his mother's kin, or in some cases both together, and participating in a ceremony which is known simply as "repairing the matter". The ceremony is conducted by a man known as a *man of akombo*, and consists of a sacrifice of chickens and goats, various small actions and repetitions of phrases performed by both the patient and the *man of akombo*, culminating in the application of medicine, mostly extract of plants, and a meal in which all the kin and spectators participate. The illness is then considered to be "repaired".

'. . . The distinctions of patient and practitioner, illness and general misfortune, are not really made by Tiv. *Akombo* means sickness but it is also used for misfortune in market, marriage, hunting and accidents. It would be true to say that for Tiv sickness is not sharply distinguished from a general run of misfortune. . . . Strictly speaking, kinfolk are held responsible for an individual's illness, and it would not be too far-fetched to consider the man's kinfolk as extended patients' (Price-Williams, 1962).

The East African Institute of Social Research held a symposium at Makerere University College, Kampala, Uganda, in December 1959, at which papers were read by social scientists on attitudes to health and disease among some African tribes. Dr L. P. Gerlach, in a paper on the Digo people of Kenya, brings out the responsibility of the kin group in two kinds of situation. When a traditional practitioner is being consulted about a sick person, his kin group has to be present at the consultation and the treatment, and the kin group assumes responsibility for paying the practitioner. If the kin group decides to take the patient to hospital, it decides who goes with the patient, who pays for his transport, and who pays for the board and lodging of the relatives who accompany the patient.

These illustrations underline the close identification of the kin group with the sick person from the onset of his illness, since the group takes decisions about treatment and participates in it. The research of social scientists in this field shows that the patient relies and is dependent on this group for support and help; and at the same time the kin group feels the illness of one of its members to be a crisis for them all, and the members' obligation and readiness to help are measures of their sense of danger to the whole group.

Disruptive elements

There is, however, another aspect of the role of the group of a person's relatives in illness. It is sometimes easy, when examining the relations between kinship groups, social structure, and ideas about disease, to overstress both the benign influence of the kinship group and its solidarity in intention and in action on behalf of someone who is ill. Many societies believe that there are potentially harmful influences working in their midst, and that these influences may operate through living persons, as well as through nature spirits or through ancestral spirits. Living individuals may be thought to be sorcerers, using evil magic to achieve some bad result, or witches possessed of some mysterious internal substance which is inimical to everyone.

Latent friction and suspicion often emerge when a crisis such as illness occurs. Then distinctions between kinsfolk and affinal relatives are clearly seen, and between the members of a male kin group and their wives taken from another group. There is even potential suspicion of the attitude of parents towards their own children, as in some African societies, where it is believed that parents can do direct harm to their children if they fail to observe the rules about intercourse after the birth of a child. Among the Ngoni, a child who is born 'too soon' after an earlier one is called 'the destroyer', because the first child does not get the mother's full attention and is weaned too soon. The disease of *kwashiorkor* is in many African societies associated with the failure of parents to observe the taboo on intercourse for a stated period after childbirth according to the cultural pattern of the society. If the parents of a child have broken this taboo, other members of the kinship group to which the children belong can accuse them of cruelty to their child and reprimand them publicly. This kind of disapproval may cause parents to try to hide a child who is suffering from the symptoms which they and their kin group associate with the syndrome called *kwashiorkor*.

In village communities where virilocal residence is the rule and the majority of wives come from outside the village and are therefore strangers, there may be an atmosphere of mistrust by the men of their stranger sisters-in-law and daughters-in-law, or even of the wives themselves by their own husbands. The writer has heard furious accusations hurled at his wife by a man who found what he thought was a queer substance, a foreign body of some kind, in the food that she had cooked for him. The episode remained in his mind, and when, later on, he or someone of his close kin did fall ill he accused this wife of having tampered with his food. On the other hand, it frequently happens that a wife does tamper with her husband's food to protect herself and her children, if he has been away on a long journey or on a spell of work in another country. Then she drops the juice of a root in the first meal she cooks for him, as a protective measure, so that, since he probably slept with other women when he was away, this intercourse with stranger women shall not harm his children or herself.

Very strict regulations imposed by the male kin group in a society may cause the women of that society to suffer a preventible illness, osteomalacia, as a result of enforced seclusion. Most cases of this disease, which is caused by lack of sunshine or a dietary deficiency of Vitamin D, occur in parts of the world where sunshine is abundant.

In a Bedouin area in the Negev Desert it was found that

'the lack of exposure to the sun of the patients is due not to the weather conditions but to the social customs prevailing in these areas, which force women to spend most of their time indoors, and when they go out to cover the whole body and face by dark clothing' (Groen *et al.*, 1962).

These Bedouin live in black tents made of goat hair. Men, youths, and children go out freely, but married women spend most of their lives in the tents, wearing a white shawl indoors, but outside a heavy black cloak completely covering the head and body, leaving the merest slit for the eyes. Eighty-five per cent of their calorie intake comes from barley or wheat bread of 100 per cent extraction flour. On the whole, their protein and Vitamin B complex is up to the standards of the National Research Council. But the diet is poor in Vitamins A and D and in calcium.

The main incidence of osteomalacia is among child-bearing women, who are sometimes immobilized by their pains, need a cane for support in walking, and cannot mount or ride a donkey. The study concluded:

'Thus the possibility has to be visualized that in addition to the clinically manifest cases, there occur among the Bedouin women many more where the deficiency of Vitamin D has produced only a sub-clinical deficiency state. Thus, osteomalacia may be, like other deficiency diseases, only the top of an iceberg the bulk of which lies under water. . . . All cases reacted, sometimes dramatically, to therapy with Vitamin D.'

CHAPTER 3

The role of the traditional practitioner

Throughout human history there has always been a place in human societies for individuals who claim to be able to give assistance in certain kinds of illness. Even in countries where professional medical care is highly developed, individual 'healers', some of them with little if any scientific training, continue to practise their real or alleged skills and to attract a clientele of people who would describe themselves as well educated. In many developing countries, among rural and largely illiterate populations, traditional practitioners commend themselves to the local community and make good their claim to possess special skills in the art of healing through their knowledge, their reputation, their personality, their relative success, and their method of approach to people who seek their aid. In societies as yet barely touched by modern medicine the kin group, as we have seen, decides whom it will consult, and, having consulted him, takes his advice about immediate action. This action may include approaching another kind of traditional practitioner or taking the sick person to a hospital or health centre.

Modern anthropological, psychological, and psychiatric research has to some extent corrected earlier and often erroneous impressions about the function and reputation of traditional practitioners. They have at times been identified exclusively with magic or witchcraft, but the way is now open for a more realistic understanding of the role they serve in their societies. The approach from the scientific medical side to these traditional practitioners and 'specialists' has come chiefly from two directions. Physicians have been interested in the knowledge and use of traditional herbal remedies, and some physicians have collected and classified these herbs, roots, and barks with the initiative and help of local herbalists and medicine men. A more recent approach to traditional practitioners has come from western-trained psychiatrists, who have studied mental ill health in developing countries and become aware of the need for prevention and treatment in conditions of increasing stress and tension.

As a result of studies by social scientists two main categories of traditional practitioner have been recognized: those who carry out treatment, the 'healers', including those who appear to heal the mentally sick as well as those suffering physically; and those who can be called 'diagnosticians'. This distinction, though convenient, is by no means a rigid one, for in some cultures and in some circumstances the diagnostician also undertakes the healing process.

TYPES OF HEALER

Health personnel and anthropologists have distinguished several kinds of healer. First, there are the women, whose skills in the use of home remedies, widespread across the world, are shared by countless others. Women's techniques include such practices as the use of purgatives and emetics, poulticing, inducing sweating by various processes, and all the traditional birth practices.

Second, there are those practitioners who learned through inheritance or apprenticeship certain manipulative skills, such as bone-setting, massage, traditional forms of vaccination, and primitive surgery. A paper to the Makerere symposium (see p. 11 above) reports that, among the Toro of Uganda, besides the doctor-diviner there are the specialist midwife and the bone-setter. The specialist midwife is called in to difficult labour cases and is an expert in administering infusions of roots and leaves to speed up delivery. The bone-setters burn the dislocated or painful joint with a red-hot nail. Some of these specialists have great reputations and are called from long distances to attend to patients.

Third, there is the best-known category, the herbalists, whose knowledge of the properties and use of herbs, roots, and barks is often very extensive. The role of diviner and herbalist was studied by physicians and botanists among the Shona and Ndebele in Rhodesia. In the Mashonaland study (Gelfand and Wild, 1955, 1959) several *nyanga* or 'doctors' cooperated to collect and name 240 specimens of herbs used in remedies for various complaints. Some of these *nyanga* were both diviners and herbalists, whereas others were only herbalists and left it to a diviner to find the cause of the illness. In the Matabeleland study (Harvey and Armitage, 1961), twenty-one *nyanga* cooperated. They chose the area for research, showed the growing herbs, explained their use for the treatment of certain symptoms, and indicated how frequently they were used. They collected 130 plants, twelve of which were used for psychical treatments. This study contains tables showing, for each plant, the botanical and Ndebele name, the dosage prescribed, and the disease for which it is considered efficacious.

Fourth, there is the category of healers who perform their healing function through a form of ritual, such as the *singer* of the Navaho, and religious leaders in other societies. Among the Navaho the term for the medicine man or healer as distinct from the diagnostician is translated as *singer*. These are the men who carry out the ceremonials designed 'to bring the dangerous under control, to drive out evil and attract the good and beautiful. One type of ceremonial, Blessing Way, protects the individual from future harm' (Adair, Deuschle, and McDermott, 1957). The preparation to become a *singer* may take several years and is learned through apprenticeship to an established *singer*. It involves learning hundreds of songs, legends about the ceremonials, and how to make sand paintings; and, in addition to the minutely accurate conduct of the ritual, many *singers* know a good deal of practical medicine, such as opening abscesses and setting bones, and applying herbal remedies.

THE DIAGNOSTICIAN–DIVINER

In some societies, preparation for the role of diviner or diagnostician is more exacting than that for the role of healer. Sometimes it is the reverse, as among the Navaho:

'When an individual falls ill and notifies his family, an informal discussion follows as to what should be done. Often they call in a diagnostician who, in a trance state, divines the cause of the illness. The most common technique is hand trembling. By what is reported to be an involuntary motion of the hand and arm, which may spread to the whole body, a finger of the hand draws symbols in the sand and rubs them out again. Eventually one will be left which will indicate the cause of the illness and what ceremony is needed to cure it. . . . Early in the research at Many Farms it was discovered that hand tremblers living in the area were advising their patients to go to the clinic in certain circumstances rather than to the medicine man' (Adair *et al.*, 1957).

In the area where the Cornell–Navaho study was made there were said to be 73 diagnosticians – 43 men and 30 women. This large number was considered to reflect the important role they play in contemporary Navaho society as those who decide between alternative means of curing. The technique of 'hand trembling' is of interest, since in other parts of the world, West Africa and India for example, diviners or priests, claiming to be possessed by a spirit or a god, show during their trance state the same characteristic of a sustained tremor either of one limb or of the whole body.

The Navaho–Cornell research team carried out a series of interviews with some of these diagnosticians, using a picture technique with questions (Adair *et al.*, 1957). In reply to the question 'What should they do?' when a picture was shown depicting a hand trembler and a patient, these were typical responses:

'It's pretty hard to say which they should do – it depends on what the trembler says. If she says a Navaho medicine man will cure it, then they have to have the *sing* first before they try the hospital. Sometimes the hospital is recommended and then they take him there right away. If he does not respond, they come back and have a *sing*. Generally one of the two works.'

'Sometimes what you do depends on the kind of sickness. If a man is sick inside – the bladder, kidney, appendicitis – the Navaho medicine man can't cure that – they have to go to hospital, maybe have an operation. If it's a taboo that's been broken, then they have a *sing* – that will cure it.'

The diagnostician is the person often consulted first by a sick person and his family, and he recommends a certain course of action to be followed to cure the patient of his complaint. In some societies such a person is called a 'diviner', and he may go into a trance and be 'possessed' by a spirit who is said to communicate to the diviner the cause of the illness and perhaps the treatment to be recommended.

Among the Ngoni of Malawi and the neighbouring peoples the writer found several categories of diviner, ranging from the prophets who foretell coming events, through those who diagnose the cause of illness, to those who deal with minor problems such as theft. Those of the first two categories are held by the Ngoni to be in very close touch with their ancestral spirits, and this is said to give them their insight and their power. They are called *abantu benhloko* – people of the head – because they see visions in their dreams, and because they live slightly apart, with their families, from general village life.

'They had all been through the experience described as *ukutwasa* – a Ngoni term signifying rebirth, and used of the reappearance of the new moon after the period of darkness. It began with physical symptoms, such as fainting, lack of appetite, forgetfulness, sweating. . . . The symptoms culminated in sharp pains and a prolonged collapse, and after that a deep sleep. It was then that the dreams came giving the man the assurance that he was thenceforth a medium, and that through the spirit of his grandfather, or another ancestor who was now appearing to him, he could communicate with the spirit world. At this time also he was told in dreams where to find medicines and what do do with them. . . . As he returned to normality from an experience which was frightening in its intensity, it dawned on him that he now had to practise as a diviner, to make use of the powers which had come to him. There was evidence that he accepted this role with reluctance. . . . Sometimes a diviner began to practise by associating as a junior partner with a successful practitioner; sometimes he began hesitantly by himself. The criterion of the validity of their calling was their success' (Read, 1956, pp. 187-8 and 198-9).

Two types of traditional practitioner among the Zulu, with whom the Ngoni have cultural links, have been described:

'The Zulu conceive of two separate kinds of medical knowledge among their own practitioners, which may be said to mirror their concepts of the two kinds of causation of disease. The herbalist, whether amateur or professional, part-time or whole-time, is known and acknowledged to have special skill in the identification and preparation of natural remedies, but this experience gains him no particular status relative to men who are skilled in any other purely technical accomplishment.

'The diviner, on the other hand, is held in the highest esteem by the Zulu, in virtue of his special knowledge of the supernatural aspects of disease and misfortune. In addition to identifying the origin of the supernatural causes of misfortunes in general, he is particularly skilled in the diagnosis and treatment of diseases held to be primarily or solely supernatural in origin. . . . Within his social context the diviner sees the total environment of the patient and his troubles much more clearly than does the Western doctor practising medicine among the Zulu. The latter cannot fail to be aware of the existence of beliefs among his patients concerning the importance of witchcraft and sorcery in causing disease; but he generally neither grasps their significance for his work nor their essentially logical nature as a theory of causation. Certainly, he does not share the beliefs with his patient.

'The diviner does all these things. His effectiveness depends very largely on his sensitive appreciation of the intricacies of personal relations in Zulu society. He is well aware of the significance of relations between social groups to the diagnosis and treatment of disease. . . .

'The diviner has a very wide field of relatively absolute expected authority, accepted by his patients in so far as he is recognised as having the necessary expertise. . . . The diviner is able to pronounce on almost any aspect of the life of his patients without risk of objections being raised. . . . There is no doubt that many Zulu patients obtain great help and relief from the emotional security involved in this surrender' (Loudon, 1957).

From Nigeria come two assessments by psychiatrists of the function of traditional practitioners:

'It would seem improper to end the subject of African traditional beliefs, concepts of health, and medical practice, without some reference to our observations on the personality structure and behavior of the native medicine men. According to our observation, some of the lesser known ones, especially on the West Coast of Africa, have proved to be either impostors or enthusiasts; their methods are either the work of a designing intellect or of an over-heated imagination. Nevertheless, a good many of them display extraordinary qualities of mind – common sense, great eloquence, great boldness, and their work displays great controversial dexterity. Generous sentiments, disinterested virtue, reverential faith, sublime speculations are the essential features of tribal medical practice. By professing to hold communion with and control supernatural beings, he can exercise an almost boundless influence over those about him.

'On the other hand, it is equally true that the well known "native therapists" employ, in addition, their knowledge of the property of herbs for the purpose of curing disease, and that they attain, in this respect, a skill which is hardly equalled by the regular practitioners' (Lambo, 1963).

The second assessment from Nigeria (Prince, 1961) refers to the distinction made by the Yoruba people in Nigeria between diviners and herbalists in respect of both role preparation and techniques. The diviners, or *babalawo*, have to memorize portions of an oral religio-medical poem of 256 chapters or verses. The diviner, when a patient and his relatives consult him, casts lots of kola nuts or cowries, and the way in which they fall indicates which verses refer to the illness or problem of the supplicant. The diviner then interprets those verses and gives the patient advice. The supplicant or patient does not tell the diviner the nature of his problem or illness because the diviner is supposed to 'know' this through his spirit contacts. It is evident, nevertheless, that in many instances the anxiety level of the patient is reduced when the diviner names the illness and explains what has caused it. The diviner assumes the responsibility of advising about personality problems as well as about the specific illness which is the object of the consultation, telling the patient to be less arrogant, to be kinder to his wife, and so on.

RELATIONSHIP WITH PATIENT AND KIN GROUP

The traditional practitioner, as he appears in recent studies by medical personnel and social scientists, is an essential link in the chain binding the patient and his kin group to the process of diagnosing and treating the illness. Local communities expect the practitioner to take a detailed and personal interest in the patient. He on his side considers it important to create an atmosphere of confidence and trust to allay the anxiety felt by the patient and his friends, and he establishes this atmosphere by an unhurried and patient question-and-answer process, as well as by the kind of inquiries he makes about the illness and its symptoms. Each symptom is considered and treated separately and not as a complex. Local practitioners are willing to be 'called' and to visit the patient in his own home, surrounded by his relatives. Even more important, the local practitioner speaks to the patient and his relatives about the illness and treatment in language and concepts that are familiar to them, and that they can understand and gratefully accept.

RELATIONSHIP WITH MODERN MEDICAL PERSONNEL

Research and experience have shown that the traditional practitioner has a potential role in modern health programmes which is recognized by some western-trained personnel. A French physician in Equatorial

Africa wrote of his experience of contacts with local medicine men, who travelled with him in his car, dressed in white coats, to help him to make contact with the villagers (Loison, 1960).

Conferences with herbalists, diviners, and shrine priests in Togoland carried out by a health educator showed that many people went to them as an outlet for their anxieties. These local practitioners might, and often did, recommend the patients to go and get modern medical treatment in a hospital. But at the same time they were providing advice and a measure of therapy on a supernatural level.

'Because certain health beliefs were strongly held throughout the region the traditional health practitioners were in a position to influence the outcome of village activities and the use made by their people of modern medical facilities. It was for this reason that, as an experiment, we arranged in five different areas three day meetings with influential herbalists, diviners, shrine priests and witchdoctors. (The selection and order of invitation was a matter of great care.) The subject for discussion was simply health and sickness, and there was no program. I was more anxious to listen than to talk, and I answered questions and discussed topics that they raised. . . . While many of them were prepared to accept the germ theory of infection they showed, of course, the familiar preoccupation with "why" does a particular man get sick rather than "how". A discussion of the multiple factors involved in disease causation was of interest to them as also was the development of modern medicine from humble beginnings. . . . They were impressed by the new drugs and admitted freely that these could cure disease that they found difficult. Nevertheless they stressed that they too were helping sick people and those in trouble. It would clearly have been useless to counter such beliefs head on; the most one could hope to do was to present modern medicine as having had its own grass roots, and as being not totally divorced from the herbalist's lore and the shrine priest's probing search for marital disharmony or kinship dispute underlying physical ills. . . . What is clear is that resort to these practitioners serves as an outlet for anxieties not confined to those created by the belief complex itself. My impression amongst those I met was that they were not unwilling to permit and even recommend modern medical treatment at the same time as they were providing advice and therapy on the supernatural level' (Spens, 1960).

The role of the traditional practitioner

Establishing contact between western physicians and Navaho medicine men was also thought to be important:

'At Many Farms from the outset we recognised the importance of working within the framework of Navaho values with respect to the curing process, both traditional and scientific. We predicted that the patients would seek out the medicine man even though they sought the help of the physicians, and this would be done (seemingly) without conflict. While the doctor could rid the body of pain and drive out the germs which he said were the cause of infection, for the religious Navaho that was not enough. The religious and psychological support of the Navaho curer was frequently needed by the patient in order to gain correct balance in the total environment. Several medicine men, at their suggestion, performed an hour-long Blessing Way ceremony at the Clinic's dedication' (Adair, 1958).

ASSOCIATIONS OF TRADITIONAL PRACTITIONERS

Traditional practitioners in some countries have shown recently that they are aware of their potential role as 'fellow-workers' with medical personnel by organizing themselves into associations. In Rhodesia it was reported that many of the *nyanga*, or medicine men, who take high fees as a rule and whose practice extends into Zambia and Malawi, are organized into the *Nyanga* Association, which gives generously to charities (Gelfand and Wild, 1955, 1959; Harvey and Armitage, 1961). In Nigeria there are several associations of traditional 'doctors', some of which hold examinations and give certificates (Prince, 1961). In Ghana the new Local Councils regard all shrine priests as private practitioners of native medicine, who have to pay several guineas a year for their licences to practise (Field, 1960).

These associations found in Africa could be regarded as a form of rearguard action against the advance of modern health programmes. They are also an attempt by traditional practitioners to rationalize their own procedures; to eliminate if possible incompetent and ill-directed efforts by individuals calling themselves medicine men; and to meet organized scientific medicine with a form of organization, recognized at least by themselves. Further research into the existence and purposes of these self-directed organizations of traditional practitioners should yield useful results for any assessment of the place of traditional knowledge and skills in the treatment of physical and mental illness.

CHAPTER 4

Traditional ideas about sickness and treatment

CATEGORIES OF ILLNESS AND TREATMENT
IN TRADITIONAL SYSTEMS

Some attempts have been made by physicians and social scientists in tropical areas to examine local traditional classifications of illness. These categories are distinguished by symptoms as recognized by the local people, and by the regions of the body and mind which are alleged to be affected in the sick person. They are also integrally related to what the people believe to be the causes of the illness.

It has been suggested by two medical workers of wide experience (Jelliffe and Bennett, 1960) that in African systems there are three groups of illnesses. The first are trivial or everyday complaints treated by home remedies. The second are 'European diseases' – that is, diseases that respond to western scientific therapy, such as yaws and malaria. The third category is of 'African diseases' – those not likely to be understood or treated successfully by western medicine. The same authors also put together a list of traditional treatments in more than one tropical area. They speak of the type of dietetic treatment in which 'hot' foods are given for 'cold' complaints, and vice versa. Physiotherapeutic treatment includes massage and poultices, and counter-irritants include cupping and scarification. Herbs are used medicinally, as in many parts of the world, and operative techniques cover cataract removal and circumcision, both male and female. For the mentally ill, to drive out the demons, use is made of beating, fasting, icy baths, or a smoke hut.

This kind of threefold classification has been suggested for other areas besides Africa. It is useful as a guide-line in seeking to understand people's attitudes towards what they recognize as illness as distinct from health, and what they expect in the way of cures or treatment from their own resources as well as from modern medicine.

In a North Indian situation a western physician (Gould, 1957) had considerable difficulty in trying to find out why the village people came to him for certain complaints and not for others. Questions based on

24

the terminology used showed that the people talk about 'country medicine' and 'doctor medicine'. They also distinguish chronic non-incapacitating illness, such as rheumatism, from critical incapacitating illness, such as typhoid, malaria being on the borderline between the two. Villagers hold that chronic illness can be treated by 'country medicine', whereas the others need 'doctor medicine'.

Many of the recent studies have been made in Latin American cultures. The concept of 'hot' and 'cold' in relation to diseases and to diet, which has become familiar from these studies, is found in many other areas also. In a study of health in a Mexican–American culture four main categories of disease were recognized (Clark, 1959). The first includes diseases due to 'hot' and 'cold' imbalance in the human body, which can be modified by 'cold' and 'hot' diets respectively. Such descriptive terms, as is well known, do not depend on the temperature of the body or of the food, and they have to be learned by health workers who are unfamiliar with the underlying cultural concepts. The second category contains diseases caused by dislocation of internal organs, such as a 'fallen fontanelle', obstruction of the gastro-intestinal tract, varicose veins. Third come diseases of magical origin, caused by the 'evil eye', when someone admires a child; or 'bad air' (*mal air*), which causes facial twisting or sometimes epilepsy; or witchcraft, which can cause barrenness. The last category covers diseases of emotional origin, due to anger, fright, or something called 'soul loss'. Much the same kinds of category have been described in Peru and Chile, with emphasis on the 'core illnesses' which are due to emotional stress, ritual uncleanness, and 'bad air'. None of these can be cured by western physicians (Simmons, 1955).

CULTURAL CONCEPTS OF HEALTH AND DISEASE

Several recent socio-medical studies reveal a deep concern with their bodily condition among people who have not had easy access to health services. In one account, a general view of the Navaho attitude is given:

'The Navaho conception of health is very different from ours. For him, health is symptomatic of a correct relationship between man and his environment: his supernatural "environment", the world around him, and his fellow man. Health is associated with good, blessing and beauty – all that is positively valued in life. Illness, on the other hand, bears evidence that one has fallen out of this delicate balance; it is usually ascribed to the breaking of one of the taboos which guide the behavior of the Navahos, especially in the case of the conservative elders. Illness may also be due to contact with the ghosts of the dead, or even to the malevolence of another Navaho who has resorted to witchery. . . . The Navaho does not make the distinction between religion and medicine that we do; for him they are aspects of the same thing. This is an important cultural fact that many workers in the health field have failed to realize; as a result, many doctors and nurses have antagonized their patients' (Adair *et al.*, 1957).

Confirmation of many of these beliefs about causes and origins of illness comes from experience in the Old World:

'In many cultures "health and illness" are inextricably connected with socially approved behavior and moral conduct, and hence such a view works as a stabilizing force and a deterrent pressing for social conformity. Anthropologists have reported that among several pre-literate societies it is deemed essential for the enjoyment of health to "have good thoughts, to avoid quarrelling and aggressive acts". In some rural areas of the Middle East, disease is believed to be caused either by failure to fulfil some religious ritual or ceremony, such as a financially able man not performing his pilgrimage, or the failure to give the promised offering to a saint. Curiously enough tuberculosis is believed to be caused by pretence and social conceit. The cultural idiom also determines the classification of diseases, the weight of their seriousness and the type of treatment required. There is "cold" illness that could be cured by medicament and there is "hot" illness that requires the placation of hidden forces. There are diseases thought to be curable by modern medicine and others thought not to be so curable, and in the light of such a division one knows what kind of "specialist" he would call' (Ammar, 1960).

An Egyptian physician says[1] that peasant people in the villages of rural Egypt believe that illness must be associated with pain and discomfort, otherwise it is not illness. Hence bilharziasis and other parasitic infections are not illness because they do not cause pain and therefore do not require treatment. The presence of mild ill health is accepted as

[1] Personal communication.

a normal part of life, and if anyone is indisposed or 'out of sorts' with such symptoms as mild fever, headache, cough, diarrhoea, he can be treated by home remedies and no outside help is sought. The main causes of illness according to the villagers are the evil eye, spirit possession, black magic, emotional strains and stresses, colds, and fever. Emotional strains can cause any type of disease. Their core is fear or sorrow, and there is a special brass decorated cup called the 'fear cup' from which a child who has been stricken by fear must drink. Cold air is the source of many complaints in the heart, bladder, kidneys, joints.

In an account of Indian village life in Hyderabad State, an anthropologist relates illness to the ritual structure of Hindu life, emphasizing that the punctilious observance of the ritual cycle of festivals leads to the prosperity and wellbeing of families:

'Most of the common diseases are interpreted as a "fault in the physical system", and are treated with herbal medicines or modern drugs obtained from the dispensary. Common colds, headaches, stomach ache, scabies, gonorrhoea and syphilis are regarded as natural diseases, and an effort is made to cure them with medicines. But persistent headaches, intermittent fevers, continued stomach disorders, rickets and other wasting diseases among children, menstrual troubles, repeated abortions, etc. are attributed to supernatural forces. In all such cases medicinal cures as well as propitiation of the "unseen powers" are attempted simultaneously. Similarly such calamities as the failure of crops, total blindness, repeated failures in undertakings, deaths of children in quick succession and too many deaths in the family within a short time, are taken to indicate "misfortune" and "the handiwork of malevolent supernatural forces". Smallpox, cholera and plague are always attributed to the wrath of various goddesses. For these diseases worship is regarded as the only remedy; and no medicines are administered to the patient' (Dube, 1955, p. 127).

Another anthropologist who has worked in North India discusses the report of a Committee on Indigenous Systems of Medicine in India, published by the Ministry of Health in 1948, which states:

'Western medicine has chiefly considered the study of disease as the result of outside agencies like the microbes. Indian medicine considers disease as a state of disharmony in the body as a whole and a result not only of the external factors nor merely of the external causes. Hence, according to it, treatment should aim at not only the finding of appropriate internal remedies, but the employment of all available means to restore the normal balance or equilibrium. The comprehensiveness of the Indian medicine is further evident from the attention it gives to diet – both in health and in disease. It takes into account not only the prevailing season and climate but also the temperament and constitution of the individual' (Opler, 1963).

He goes on to summarize the view of sickness and its proper treatment as he studied it in the rural areas of eastern Uttar Pradesh. Good health consists of the proper functioning of three factors in the human body, wind, bile, and phlegm, and the malfunctioning of any one results in a specific ailment. In many cases the imbalance and sickness are due to faulty diet, and can be adjusted by strict nutritional controls, including preliminary fasting. Immoderation or inappropriate behaviour in physical, social, and even economic matter is not without danger to bodily health. One famous Ayurvedic doctor in the area was known to be very severe with patients who in his opinion had weakened their bodies by sexual excesses. Lack of harmony with the supernatural world can bring on sickness, and so can the activities of aggrieved and unrequited ghosts.

Opler concludes by emphasizing the significance of protective ritual:

'Many standard rites are in fact precautionary ceremonies in which a deity is regularly honored, so that he will bear his worshippers good will only. For example, just before the season when smallpox is likely to erupt, a rite in honor of the Smallpox Goddess is carried out in each household, in the course of which she is fed, honored and ceremonially led from the vicinity.'

A medical psychiatrist and anthropologist, writing about the Hindu Body Image, added another factor to these descriptions of beliefs about illness in North India:

'While they were sick, my patients felt themselves to be invaded by something evil. This might be expressed in physical terms, as bad air, bad blood, or phlegm; but still more often it was personified, as the invasion of one's body by a witch or evil spirit. The crisis of a cure always coincided with the summoning of this spirit, and its

28

being exorcised with bribes or threats. Once this was done, the patient might feel weak, but he knew his life was saved; from now on he could look forward to recovery' (Carstairs, 1957, p. 83).

ILLNESS AND BEHAVIOUR

An anthropologist, physician, and clinical psychiatrist, with extensive previous knowledge of Ghana, made a study of the rural shrines and their place in the health and sickness practices of the people (Field, 1960). In the undefined field between physical illness and mental illness, the research is of special significance. In the preface to her study she says:

'I found that the shrines, particularly in Ashanti, were still multiplying, and that they were still the first resort of people who had become in any way mentally ill, whether trivially or gravely. . . . The picture of mental illness seen by the rural field worker must be essentially different from that seen by the Mental Hospital Psychiatrist. The rural patient is never taken to the mental hospital, not because of any associated stigma, but because the illness is regarded as supernaturally determined and hence outside the province of hospitals.'

After describing the socio-economic background of the people, their ideological background, and the phenomena associated with spirit possession, she analyses the troubles and desires of ordinary people, as they appear in their recourse to the shrines. The close connexion between illness and behaviour, found also in India and Egypt and among the Navaho, is plain:

'At the shrine the possessed priest questions the supplicant as he does those who complain simply of physical sickness, and if he elicits family strife and anxiety he advises concerning it. . . . Organic illness is almost always attributed to either witchcraft, bad medicine, or sin, seldom to worry or stress. . . . Although the shrine therapists recognize their limitations and frequently tell patients with pneumonia, cardiac failure or pulmonary distress with blood coughing, to go to the hospital, they stand firmly on the theory that the primary vulnerability of the patient to the disease is of supernatural origin, and until redemptive ritual has been performed the hospital efforts are futile. . . . When a sick child is brought to the shrine the priest invariably seeks first for strife between the parents, a circumstance in which, it is held, no young child can thrive. . . . Though the commonest reason assigned for the sickness of a child is open quarrelling between the parents, a number of mothers were blamed for adultery, refusal of intercourse with the father, and plain neglect of the child. . . . Again a child may be a bone of contention between its father and its mother's brother (the latter being, in a matrilineal system, its next of kin and sometimes over-possessive), and this again is held to spoil the child's well-being' (Field, 1960).

EXAMPLES OF BELIEFS AND PRACTICES

Some African tribal groups

The ideas of several East African tribal peoples concerning the causes of illness and appropriate treatment are described below. The first four accounts are taken from papers presented at the Makerere symposium in 1959.

A mountain people, *the Sebei, on Mt Elgon in Kenya,* give causes and categories of disease, most of them associated with specific illnesses:

Causes and categories of disease	*Associated illnesses*
Ancestor spirits	Eye and ear diseases
Spells of wizards	General weakness
Rainbow 'from above'	Miscarriages, children's illnesses
Wrongdoing, evil eye	Fever, stomach pains
Killing a man	Madness
Hereditary clan diseases	Epilepsy, skin lesions, swellings, and sores
Common everyday complaints	Colds, malaria, eye disease, swellings

The Digo people in Kenya have a tendency to hypochondria, and are very interested in the subject of health and disease. They spend considerable time, effort, and wealth in attempting to maintain or to restore good health. They attribute disease to the following causes:

God
Ancestral spirits
Possession by evil spirits:
  these *shaitani* are responsible for hysterical behaviour; possession by these spirits affects the full range of Digo behaviour, including agriculture, business, religion, education.
Sorcery
Broken taboos
Disharmony with the supernatural:
  affecting particularly fertility, and related to pre-Islamic rites.

These same Digo people have a wide knowledge of herbal medicines, and some 50 per cent of all the men and women are 'doctors' of herbal medicines, though only 15 per cent of them are famous outside their kinship group. Koranic medicines and amulets are used, as are also patent medicines bought in the stores made up from European or Indian formulae. The belief is prevalent that medicines given in hospital are 'watered down' and therefore ineffective. After trying herbal, Koranic, and patent remedies the Digo may still go and consult a mobile dispensary if there is one in their area.

They avoid certain foods during certain illnesses, for example, salty foods during influenza. They believe, however, that the best treatment is preventive. Illness can be avoided chiefly through strict observance of the taboos on certain kinds of sexual behaviour; through wearing amulets regularly; not working on Fridays; and using proper latrines, whose possession is a source of pride to householders. This concept of preventive action to avoid ill health is widespread and arises from their views on how illness is caused and what the positive elements are in good health.

The Nyamwezi in western Tanganyika have extensive categories of illness which they express both in general terms, such as 'to be ill' and 'to get better', and more specifically as states of illness denoted by name according to symptoms: those with fever shivering, those with stabbing pains like pleurisy, those with stomach pains like worms, those with swellings like *kwashiorkor*. Then there are names for definite illnesses such as leprosy, yaws, smallpox, syphilis. There are, in addition, categories of 'public' illness such as epidemics of cholera or influenza. These are called 'God's business', as are also drought and famine. On the other hand, there are 'private and hereditary' illnesses like leprosy or elephantiasis, about which questions are asked during marriage negotiations – 'Does your family suffer from . . .?' The people consult a diviner as to the nature and cause of the disease, and he either orders a sacrifice to the ancestors or gives medicines such as roots, leaves, or parts of animals. The heart of an antelope can be given to cure madness. Aches and pains are relieved by cupping, and by incisions made on the body with medicine rubbed in. As prophylactics, charms are worn. Vaccination from a person with slight smallpox was formerly practised. And today patent medicines such as liniments and aspirins are bought in the shops.

The Samburu people in Kenya are said to have a general high standard of health and to be on the whole well nourished on a basic diet of milk. There is, however, a high infant mortality rate, and parents take special care of children in their early years. They have a horror of 'inner' and ritual uncleanness, and consider that disease is a sort of poison which can be expelled by purgatives. They use medicinally a wide range of plants and trees, many of which are purgatives and emetics, others stimulants. Their positive concept of health is to keep the body system clear through taking purgatives, and by avoiding contact with any form of excrement, which they consider as most unclean. Eggs are regarded as hens' excrement, and therefore avoided. Other unclean foods include fish, donkey, dog, elephant, bush pig, monkey. They carry this revulsion from uncleanness so far that they do not like to marry women from certain tribes that eat unclean food. This same horror extends to the fact and idea of death, and after a funeral there are elaborate cleansing ceremonies.

The Somali (Brotmacher, 1955), who set a high value on milk as a food, treat illnesses according to the symptoms as recognized by the *wadad* or local practitioner. He treats anaemia with lightly cooked liver, other complaints with milk diet or infusions of rice, with poultices, cauterization, and bleeding. Sterility is treated with a high fat diet and with applications of pounded roots. The Somali have practised a form of vaccination from an infected smallpox case, and 25 per cent were found thus vaccinated in a survey of 1,000. This form of vaccination has been found elsewhere in East Africa.

Traditional ideas about sickness and treatment

The Sukuma people in north-west Tanganyika (Tanner, 1959), who practise animal husbandry and agriculture, have an enormous pharmacopoeia of some thousands of plants. Their knowledge of medicine and minor surgery is not, as in some other areas, confined to the specialist class of diviners and magicians, but is widespread over the whole population. The basis for their classification of disease is a description of physical symptoms, but there are no exclusive categories attributable to one particular cause. The medicines and treatments that they use include cupping, incisions, and splints; steaming, snuffing, and plasters on the chest for coughs; infusions of herbs, and herbs in cooked food. These 'cures', however, are only a part of the complete treatment advocated, which in the majority of cases is largely spiritual.

The Eskimo

Among the Eskimo (Lantis, 1959), folk medicine and hygiene include treatment for illness and some traditional preventive practices to make people strong. Their rigorous environment demands a maximum knowledge and use of all possible therapeutic devices. Heated leaves are used to relieve joint pains, and tisanes for internal pains in the stomach and intestines, including willow-bark infusions which contain salicylic acid. [A fungus is boiled to make a laxative; cranberry juice is applied for snow blindness; and resin and sphagnum moss are used to cover wounds. From their animals they use fats, oils, and blood for medicaments, and also blood, saliva, milk, and urine from their own bodies. Urine was formerly used to stop wounds bleeding, warm seal-oil to treat earache, and seal-oil and urine as laxatives.

Thermal treatment includes sweat baths and the application of hot stones or ashes or leaves for arthritis. Snow or ice are used to stop nosebleeding. Acupuncture and blood-letting are practised with a special needle and great skill. On the preventive side, cleaning of the body was done with boys' urine, which was held to be good for removing oil and dirt, and by sweat baths. Young people were made to take special exercises, and severe control was exercised over eating, drinking, and hours of sleeping.

Attitudes towards smallpox in India

A pilot survey in connexion with a health education programme on smallpox in North India (Bharara, 1961) disclosed a variety of beliefs regarding the cause of this disease:

33

Cause	% believing
The Goddess Mata	55·8
Unseen living organism	19·2
Unknown	16·7
Evil spirits	3·6
Foul smells	2·3

In the same area 45·4 per cent of the people had had experience of small-pox in their own homes, and they had acted in the following way in consequence:

Action taken	% people
Stopped all frying of food and taking of condiments	67·5
Stopped combing hair	66·8
Stopped shaving hair	48·5
Worshipped Goddess Mata in the village	56·1
Worshipped Goddess Mata in the home	44·3
Made sacrificial offerings to Goddess Mata	22·7
Stopped all work	37·6
Gave no treatment to the patient	41·2

CROSS-CULTURAL UNDERSTANDING AND COMMUNICATION

The material from many countries illustrates the great variety of concepts about the symptoms and causes of illness, which have resulted in traditional methods of diagnosis and treatment, older than, but now coexistent with, modern scientific medicine. There are instances of the connexion between illness and 'behaviour', and between health and harmony, which can be understood only in terms of cultural patterns and social relationships. This understanding is made more difficult where language barriers exist between the western-trained health worker and the local people.

The language barrier and problems of conceptual transfer

Overcoming the language barrier was an important aspect of the research carried out in the Navaho–Cornell experiment. It was found, when training Navaho health visitors at the clinic, that the Navaho have an extensive terminology for the skeletal system but virtually none for the circulatory and nervous systems. Moreover, in an anatomical laboratory demonstration, when a sheep was dissected, and the similarity between sheep and human organs pointed out, it was found that the Navaho have only one word for the thoracic cavity contents, because when they kill a sheep they remove all these organs *en masse*. Hence new Navaho words had to be found for trachea, heart, lungs, etc.

On the question of how physicians can adjust to language problems in medical aid programmes, it was concluded:

> 'If the physician shows an interest in language at a general social level, and can acquire a few phrases helpful in directing or greeting persons in the clinic, he can establish good rapport with his patients. In order to utilize the full benefits of his scientific training across a formidable cultural and language barrier, such as exists with tribal people, it is better for the physician to learn the principles of conceptual transfer and spend the necessary time training his interpreters and himself in the medical concepts of the two cultures. When he is acquainted with the cultural matters involved in the particular change, he is far less apt to overlook the intensive questioning of an area of importance' (Deuschle, 1963).

In another article on the same study this problem of conceptual transfer, as the physicians met it in the field, is further explained:

> 'The problem of physician–patient communication with Navaho people is a formidable one, not so much because there are wide differences between the Navaho and the English language as because there are wide differences between the two cultures with respect to concepts of bodily disease. If both cultures had essentially the same concepts of disease and its treatment, any person reasonably fluent in both languages could serve as a satisfactory "bridge" between the patient and his physician. As it stands, however, with the wide difference in medical concepts that exist, an interpreter may be completely bilingual in discussing the ordinary affairs of life yet wholly unreliable in discussing medical matters unless he is quite generally familiar with the medical concepts of both cultures. To be sure, this same principle applies in some degree to technologies other than medicine. But in most other technologies – for example animal husbandry or agriculture – the two people involved in the attempt at communication are both usually concerned with the visible world around them and not with the inner feelings of one of the two persons.

By contrast, for the proper application of modern medicine the physician depends to a very considerable extent (exclusively, for some diseases) on the subtleties and minor gradations in the patient's own account of how he feels as compared with his usual state.

'Thus, in the case of the Navaho, the patient's own standards, by which he judges his degree of well-being, are not only not known to the physician but they derive from concepts of whose very existence the physician may be unaware' (McDermott *et al.*, 1960).

A similar area of linguistic confusion for scientifically trained health personnel is the range of words with which a patient discusses pain. He attempts to describe pain in a particular region of the body; the kind of pain he feels, whether dull, aching, sharp, or stabbing; and the intensity of pain up to the point of its being unbearable. In some societies people are trained from childhood to endure pain or even to deny its existence. Some recent midwifery studies bring this out. There are societies where a woman in labour must never utter a sound, however intense her pain may be. She will even deny the existence of pain when questioned by the midwife, sometimes because the occurrence of difficult labour is considered in some cultures to be due to the woman's infidelity to her husband.

Standard dictionaries of local languages can at times lead western physicians astray, as shown by the following example of linguistic confusion over the concept underlying the malnutrition syndrome known as *kwashiorkor*:

'When Digo note the syndrome of *kwashiorkor* in a child they state he is suffering from *chirwa*. *Chirwa* is the passive form of a verb which is used in the sense of doing something very wrong – i.e. to break a taboo. *Chirwa* cannot in any way be translated as illness resulting from malnutrition. Digo have no term for or concept of malnutrition. They believe that *chirwa* is the result of the transgression of a number of basically sexual taboos by the parents of the child. . . . Digo feel that if adults break a sexual taboo they will often not be punished directly, but their children will be injured by vaguely defined and conceptualized supernatural forces. . . . Because of the *chirwa* concept, Digo are reluctant to take individuals suffering from *kwashiorkor* to western medical personnel. For one thing they do not like to admit that their children have this affliction since it indicates that they have broken the taboo. . . . The standard Swahili–English dictionary used by European administrators in East Africa defines *chirwa* simply as "rickets". Europeans . . . sometimes tour Digo and other coastal locations and ask to examine children suffering from *chirwa*, and it is small wonder that few cases are made known to them' (Gerlach, 1961).

The barrier of language related to concepts of illness appears formidable to physicians and health personnel, even when they share the same spoken language as their patients, and in intercultural situations it is obviously still more difficult. Not only are patients unable to describe their symptoms adequately but they in turn often cannot understand the instructions given to them by the physician and nurse. This is particularly the case in the diagnosis and treatment of mental illness.

PART II

Social groups, culture patterns, and health

CHAPTER 5

The human group and its integration

CONTRAST BETWEEN HOSPITALIZATION AND TREATMENT IN TRADITIONAL SETTING

To the nurse and physician in a rural hospital a new patient being admitted is an individual needing the skilled attention which they alone can give him. They may or may not be aware that the sick person is afraid to deliver himself into their hands, and that he parts most reluctantly from the group of relatives and friends who have accompanied him to the hospital. It is they who have been taking care of him hitherto and have taken the decision to resort to western medicine. But, as a social scientist working in the Kentucky mountain region has pointed out (Pearsall, 1962), where illness is traditionally handled by involving the entire family, hospitalization represents a traumatic break from intimate personal support in familiar surroundings to impersonal attention from professionals in a strange and forbidding environment. As another anthropologist puts it:

'In the non-hospital therapeutic relationship the patient has considerable freedom of choice: he can follow or disobey the physician's instructions, or terminate the relationship at will. But in the hospital he is at the mercy of strange and often impersonal forces, and he can no longer exercise the veto. Hospital practices conflict at important points with folk and primitive medical belief and practice, and with the sociological setting of curing. Family and friends can be near only for short periods; foods thought to be dangerous are forced on one, and evil effects may follow' (Foster, 1958, p. 25).

This reluctance to enter hospital because it means separation from the protective group is found in many rural areas:

'Cultural norms are also reflected in the resistance to hospitalization and isolation in cases of epidemics. Taking the sick to the isolation ward is considered in certain cultures as not isolating an ill man and thus preventing the infection of others, rather it is taken as a rejection of a member of the family whose responsibility and care lie primarily on his kinship group. In cases of hospitalization the regulation of visits to the sick is a frustrating experience to both the sick and his relatives. Many popular songs in Egypt express the emotional security and the sense of pride that a sick man derives from being surrounded by his family and people. One of the songs, for example, imagines a conversation between a doctor and a sick person, where the doctor asks who is going to pay for the medicine. The sick person is shocked by such a question and instantly replies that he has so many "people" who will see to it. The song goes on to show how each member of the family offers the doctor something in turn. But in the end the patient dies, because he is so aggravated and embittered by the doctor's question, which implied that he had no people to attend to him in such a matter as paying the doctor's fees and medicine charges. "To have no people" is one of the greatest insults that could be directed to any person' (Ammar, 1960, p. 13).

TWO SIGNIFICANT SOCIAL FEATURES OF RURAL LIFE

Hospitalization with its attendant fears is only one aspect of the dependence of a sick person on his social group. The health worker whose life has been spent in urban surroundings and who has been trained in an urban hospital needs reorientation in two important directions in order to grasp the significance of the family and community background to the physical and mental health of rural people.

The importance of the wider kin group

In the first place, his concept of a 'family' is usually limited to the small circle of immediate relatives belonging to the nuclear family which is characteristic of most new and many old urban settlements. Hence the terms father, mother, brother, sister have to him restricted connotations and express a limited kinship relationship rather than a complex of mutual obligations and services. The wider group of kin, referred to earlier as taking responsibility for a sick person, includes 'classificatory' fathers, mothers, brothers, grandparents, and so on, and constitutes a social group in a rural community which eludes the customary definition of a family.

The 'wholeness' of village life

The second direction in which health workers need reorientation is towards understanding the people's attitude to their life in their village as a 'whole'. Modern administration and welfare programmes operating from above divide village life into segments, such as agriculture, food habits, sanitation, child health, etc. This is not how village people regard their daily life and activities. The concept of the integration of social relationships and cultural ways of living is inherent in the anthropologist's 'holistic' approach to a community, and bears directly on the response of rural people to public health programmes and to community welfare programmes of all kinds. This and the succeeding chapters in Part II illustrate different facets of this holistic approach and the contribution it can make to the main theme of the book.

Anthropologists have been trained to use in their fieldwork several techniques for recognizing and analysing different groups in the structure of a society. The primary factor in these analyses is kinship in all its many aspects. In what are sometimes called the 'very simple societies', such as hunters and collectors in isolated environments like tropical forests or the Arctic, kinship may be virtually the only principle on which groups exist and regulate the life of the people. In most societies, individuals who have kinship ties through descent are linked with affinal relatives through marriage, and they have other relationships created by common residence in a compound, a hamlet, a village, or a neighbourhood. They are bound by mutual economic interests, including ownership of land or property, and by the pursuit of similar occupations; by religious affiliation and participation in ceremonies and ritual; by political loyalties and identification with political parties. And these are only a few of the major bonds uniting individuals in groups, and distinguishing one group from another.

AN ANTHROPOLOGIST'S APPROACH TO THE STUDY OF A MALAWI VILLAGE AND HAMLET

It may be of use to see how one anthropologist presented an analysis of some of the groups in a particular Malawi village. The writer was interested in the processes of social and economic change, which included changes in food habits and the effects of migration from the

43

villages to and from towns. The village, and the adjoining hamlet, are in an area where two culture groups organized on different social principles live side by side.

Kinship and other groups

Figures 1 and *2*[1] (pp. 46, 47) show the differences in kinship grouping between patrilineal and matrilineal families, and the differences in the roles played and the responsibilities assumed by the various kinship and affinal groups. They also illustrate how a single individual – EGO – is a member of all these groups, each of which regulates his life in respect of the roles played by the group. The patrilineal or matrilineal principle of organization emphasizes one main difference between the two culture groups. Among the patrilineal Ngoni a girl on her marriage keeps her clan name and membership of the patrilineage of her father, but exchanges her 'house' and extended family for that of her husband, and as a rule leaves the village. Among the matrilineal Cewa, however, it is the man who leaves the village on marriage, keeping the name of his name group and his personal membership of his matrilineage, but exchanging his extended family for that of his wife, in whose village he settles, and where his children 'belong'.

Activities, journeys, contacts

Figure 3 (p. 48), which refers only to the Ngoni village, illustrates what a physician in North Borneo described as a 'valuable practice' for health workers – namely, observing the activities, journeys, and contacts of the people in a village. The Ngoni combine their original political overlordship of a wide area with a considerable amount of entrepreneurship in the organization of labour in cotton and tobacco gardens, and the marketing of cattle, tobacco, and cotton. The mission station and the Indian stores are a ready market where the women sell milk, eggs, and fowls. Rather than consume these foods themselves, which they like and appreciate, most households prefer the ready cash, which

[1] *Figures 1, 2,* and *3* were used as teaching material in an American graduate seminar studying anthropological aspects of culture change, and in particular the patterns of authority in changing cultures. The diagrams are only a small part of a much larger mass of descriptive material, including genealogies of all the village families and the current habitat of all their members, which throw much light on intra-village and inter-village relationships through marriage and divorce, and on economic activities and emigration.

44

they can convert into blankets, cloth for women's garments, men's and children's clothes, shoes, equipment such as hoes and axes, salt, which is always needed, and sugar and tea, which, to some extent among the younger people, have replaced beer for entertaining friends.

A three months' record of some twenty-five households in the Ngoni village shows that, in addition to the buying and selling in stores and markets, there is a continuous interchange between the households of small loans and gifts of foodstuffs of all kinds. Many gifts also come from other villages, especially from the present Chief's village on richer soil, and from the families of the women who have married into the village, for no mother ever visits her daughter's and son-in-law's home empty-handed. It is evident from the record of these exchanges that they introduce some diversity in the day-to-day and month-to-month food habits of most Ngoni households. Money is seldom spent on food, except for such items as salt, sugar, and tea, and basically the diet depends on cultivated cereal crops. But loans here and gifts there, especially of vegetables and fowls, relieve the monotony of the basic cereal foods. From the point of view of maintaining close relationships within kinship and affinal groups, these occasional exchanges of food are an important link.

There is a heavy emigration of young Ngoni and Cewa men from the area, especially those with some schooling, to the industrial and municipal centres in south Malawi and Rhodesia. On their return, not only do they bring money and presents for a wide circle of relatives, who in return kill goats and fowls to celebrate their homecoming, but they talk about their life in the cities, and especially about the food they have had there. This makes the village women, particularly the younger ones, want to emulate these urban standards of living, while at the same time they despair of doing so with their very limited local resources.

THE RELEVANCE OF THIS APPROACH
FOR HEALTH PERSONNEL

What would a health worker get from such an analysis of kinship groups and inter-village contacts as presented in this Ngoni material?

Patterns of authority in village groups
He would first of all see that he is not just dealing with small individual independent families as he knows them in a city or in a foreign culture.

45

Figure 1   NGONI KINSHIP GROUPING IN MSUNDUZERA VILLAGE

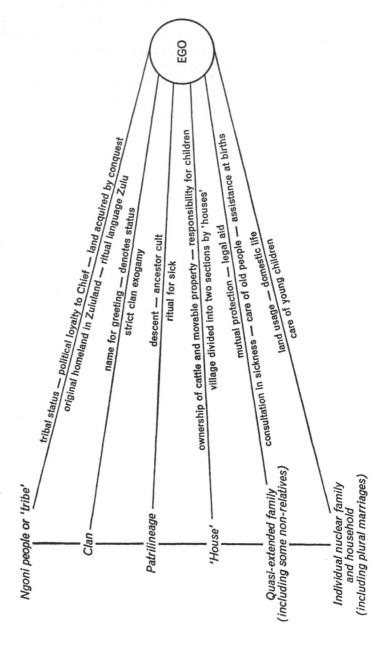

EGO

Ngoni people or 'tribe'
tribal status — political loyalty to Chief — land acquired by conquest
original homeland in Zululand — ritual language Zulu

Clan
name for greeting — denotes status
strict clan exogamy

Patrilineage
descent — ancestor cult
ritual for sick

'House'
ownership of cattle and movable property — responsibility for children
village divided into two sections by 'houses'

Quasi-extended family
(including some non-relatives)
mutual protection — legal aid — assistance at births
consultation in sickness — care of old people
land usage — domestic life
care of young children

Individual nuclear family
and household
(including plural marriages)

Figure 2   CEWA KINSHIP GROUPING IN TENJE HAMLET ADJACENT TO MSUNDUZERA

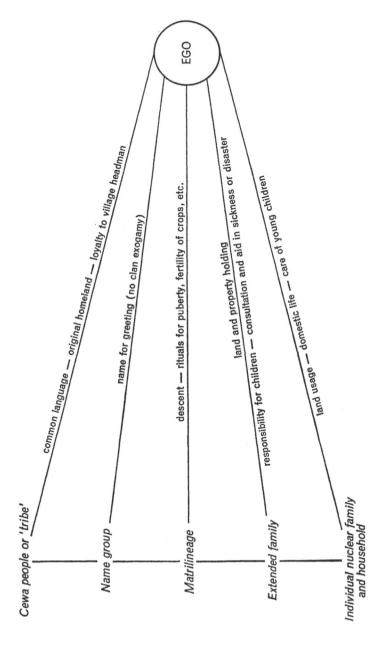

E

Cewa people or 'tribe'

common language — original homeland — loyalty to village headman

Name group

name for greeting (no clan exogamy)

Matrilineage

descent — rituals for puberty, fertility of crops, etc.

Extended family

land and property holding
responsibility for children — consultation and aid in sickness or disaster

Individual nuclear family
and household

land usage — domestic life — care of young children

EGO

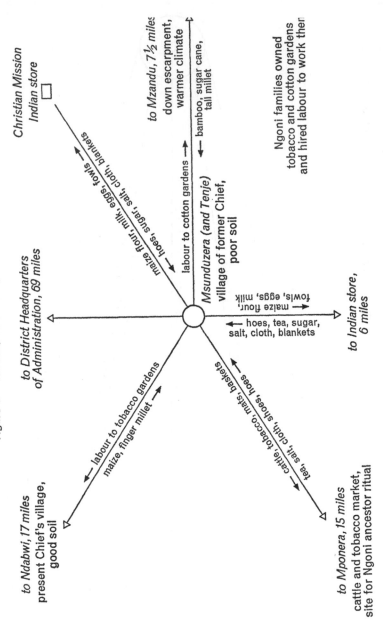

Figure 3   TRADE, MARKETS, AND LABOUR

Christian Mission
Indian store

to Mzandu, 7½ miles
down escarpment,
warmer climate

← bamboo, sugar cane,
tall millet

Ngoni families owned
tobacco and cotton gardens
and hired labour to work them

hoes, sugar, milk, eggs, cloth, blankets →
maize flour, salt, fowls →

labour to cotton gardens →

Msunduzera (and Tenje)
village of former Chief,
poor soil

maize flour,
fowls, eggs, milk →

← hoes, tea, sugar,
salt, cloth, blankets

to Indian store,
6 miles

to District Headquarters
of Administration, 69 miles

← labour to tobacco gardens
maize, finger millet →

← cattle, tobacco, mats, baskets
tea, salt, cloth, shoes, hoes →

to Ndabwi, 17 miles
present Chief's village,
good soil

to Mponera, 15 miles
cattle and tobacco market,
site for Ngoni ancestor ritual

He is dealing with a series of integrated groups, whose roles include legal responsibility for children; the disposal of property, including cattle, to find cash to pay a 'diviner' to diagnose sickness or to pay for medicines at the clinic; the care of old people, providing them with food and clothes; consultation on what kind of help to summon in case of illness or accident; care of the husband's female relatives among the Ngoni, and of the wife's maternal relatives among the Cewa; attending to births – and so on. He would find that there was a traditional pattern of authority for taking decisions on every sort of problem, from killing a bullock as a sacrifice to the ancestors when an important person was ill, to authorizing vaccination for children and deciding to take to hospital a woman in difficult labour.

Variability in food consumption

The health worker with a nutrition programme to put across would be baffled by the irregularity of the groups that eat together and by frequent changes in the food consumed due to the elaborate system of exchanges. He could argue that the women should give their children the eggs and milk that they sell, but in that case he would have to tell the women what they could do to find ready cash to buy clothes for their families. He would find that he was not the only person who had new ideas about food, but that householders gathered new ideas from the shelves in the Indian stores, from the men's talk of what food they had eaten in the towns, and from advertisements in newspapers.

Integration and disintegration in village groups

He would find too, as he observed village life more closely, that there is an atmosphere of continual activity in the village, and at certain seasons a considerable amount of coming and going to and from the village, and this does not predispose the villagers to give much time to listen to a newcomer and his plans. If he were able to stay longer in the village he might find that there is a quiet, but not very obvious, challenge to the traditional authority of the older people of high status, and that younger educated men and women sometimes take the initiative, but seldom at the expense of appearing not to 'respect' the senior people and thereby causing friction between groups. The Ngoni set a high value on 'staying together' and on not breaking up families or villages, with special emphasis on the patrilineal units, with their male leaders showing a united front. This tendency, combined with the

49

traditional respect for seniority in age and status, exercises a conservative influence on maintaining social cohesion, but leaves the way open for economic changes.

Health personnel may well argue that, unlike the anthropologist, they have no time to investigate, observe, and analyse the kinds of social group that form the structure of a given society. They can be aided, however, by the basic studies of social structures which have already been done in different parts of the world (as, for example, the series in the Ethnographic Survey of Africa directed by the International African Institute). Though the outlines of social structure in these areas are already known and form a useful starting-point, they need checking to take account of subsequent social and economic changes in the areas. The change from joint family living to individual family households or from polygamy to monogamy, the spread of modern education, and the redistribution of wealth may alter the relationship between groups and diminish the effective authority of the older members of a kin group.

The health worker needs, then, a general idea of the social structure of a particular society and the lines on which groups are organized according to kinship, marriage, residence, occupation, and status. In addition, he needs to know what activities these groups perform together; how social, economic, and religious demands – the traditional integrating elements in a society – unite different individuals for distinct and limited purposes. There are also indigenous forms of disintegration – divorce and the breaking-up of marriages; factions between rival leaders and their followers; the widening gulf in outlook and behaviour between the younger educated generation and the older traditionalists. There are many accounts of community development programmes being shipwrecked on the rocks of village factions and group rivalries. And there are societies where village groups have been held together by former rigid bonds of class or caste distinctions, where the mutual services performed by the members of one group for another have in the past sustained interpersonal links which can weaken or suddenly snap at the onset of economic or political change.

Examples from India and the Pacific

Thus a pilot study made in 1959 of health services in the Ramanagram area of Mysore reports that there are very few villages that cannot be reached by road, and that improved transport has caused many men to seek employment in the towns, so that the former static rural economy is turning into a dynamic one. This has its effect on the social organization of the village, for village solidarity has been largely undermined, and the well-integrated village structure is becoming a thing of the past.

On the other hand, another observer (Spillius, 1962) emphasizes the enduring stability of the social structure in the Pacific island of Tonga. He refers to the formal structure as being made up of a national government of a western type; nobles and executive officers; village meetings; and *kava* drinking groups. This formal structure, he says, is effective in imparting information, for example on health education programmes. It is matched by an informal structure based on kinship. News spreads through kinship channels, and every Tongan is in close touch with about fifty relatives and in less intimate touch with 100, among whom his or her father's sister has the greatest authority and the highest rank and is consulted on all matters relating to health. Villagers expect local leaders to evaluate any proposed change on their behalf. The leaders on their side do not introduce any change unless they know that the people really want it, do not require too much persuasion to adopt it, and approve of it when they see it working.

CHAPTER 6

Culture patterns and human groups

When anthropologists speak of culture, they widen and deepen the usual meaning of the term, defining the culture of a particular group as the way of living of the people in that group. It can be peculiar to them; it can have affinities with neighbouring groups; it can be a subcultural group within a larger one. The Navaho speak of living in the 'Navaho way' and contrast it with the 'white way', meaning by the latter the American culture. Within Hindu culture there are many subcultures, characteristic of economic classes and social castes, and of different geographical and ecological areas. Two Bantu-speaking peoples in Africa may, like the village groups in Malawi in the preceding chapter, share a common language and possess a common habitat, but their cultures may vary in such fundamental aspects as reckoning descent and inheritance on a patrilineal or a matrilineal basis, the significance of cattle as property, the forms of the ancestor cult, and the close integration of kinship groups and political authority.

WORKING IN AN ALIEN CULTURE

What are the most important factors to be borne in mind when health workers have to work with people who possess a different culture?

Ethnocentrism and the transfer of cultural expectations

In the first place it is useful to remember that most people are ethnocentric in their first contacts with and approaches to an alien way of living:

'To most men and women the way of life of their community is its most precious possession. To outsiders who have their own habits and assumptions, this way of life or culture often appears incongruous and misguided' (Burton, 1961).

Physicians, nurses, sanitarians, health educators often transfer from their own cultural background their expectations of how people will

52

behave or ought to behave in certain crises or conditions of illness. The scientifically trained health worker, wherever he may be, belongs to a culture, to a way of living and thinking that often has more in common with similarly trained health workers in other countries than with the illiterate rural population of his own country. Ethnocentrism has to be given a wide interpretation in order that it may be recognized as a formidable barrier to communication in public health work.

Foundations of cultural conformity

The second factor is closely related to this one. People living in their own cultural group are most of the time unaware of having a culture. They share the way of life of everyone else and can anticipate to a large extent how other people will behave. In other words, conformity to a cultural pattern ensures a large measure of predictability in behaviour. Only when individuals go outside their culture and mix with people from other cultures do they become aware of their own way of living as distinct from another way. This relative unawareness of their cultural pattern by members of a social group within their own society sometimes conceals from outsiders the fact that cultural rules and cultural behaviour are a reality in people's lives, and profoundly influence their thought and action. Cultural behaviour has to be learned, as speech and language are taught and learned, in childhood, in the home. People are not born with instinctive cultural habits. They are born *into* a culture, and from an early age they have to learn how to conform to its codes by adjusting their personal inclinations in order to live harmoniously with their relatives and neighbours. This process of learning about how to behave within one's own culture is a universal phenomenon, but people seeing a new culture or subculture from the outside often do not appreciate the effectiveness and deep roots of the learning process.

Variability in culture change

The third factor has been noted by anthropologists in several parts of the world: that social structure and social relationships change more slowly than do other aspects of culture, such as agricultural practices, economic forms of exchange, fashions in clothing and housebuilding, and so on. The health worker whose programme is aimed at changing people's cultural habits in child care, diet, or sanitation may be brought up sharply against a refusal to alter a cultural habit because it will offend a deep-rooted social relationship or a tenaciously held religious conviction. These aspects of culture change, illustrating the problems inherent when modern practices are superimposed on traditional culture patterns, call for intensive study both before and during the adoption of new health programmes. They are involved in the ambivalence towards health programmes discussed in Part III.

Awareness of culture patterns

The fourth factor is one of the major problems for health workers faced with a complex and unfamiliar way of living in a community: namely, how to see what relationships exist between the various aspects of a culture – for example agricultural practices, water usage, food habits, care of young children, and so on. The tendency is for outsiders, especially those charged with a programme for improving living conditions, to see only a series of 'customs', in particular those more obvious ones which do not tally with the outsider's cultural way of living, and which may appear as 'cultural blocks' to the implementation of the health programme. In the final section of his book, *Health, Culture and Community* (1955, p. 460), Dr Benjamin Paul reminds us that it is hard for specialists such as professional health workers to recapture the unspecialized way of seeing things, and hence it is difficult to give them an adequate grasp of the meaning of culture. Anthropologists, he says, have worked out the concept of culture as an organizing frame for encompassing the details that make up the life of a community. He maintains that the systematic features of culture are discoverable, and that what is called a pattern of culture expresses a cultural coherence to the people sharing that culture which can be, but is not always, perceived by those seeing it from the outside.

The rest of this chapter illustrates the importance of this concept of culture for understanding how people react to modern health programmes.

THE CULTURAL SIGNIFICANCE OF FOOD HABITS

It may be difficult to assert that any one facet of a people's culture is more vital than another in conditioning their beliefs and practices about health and disease. Yet it is generally accepted that the cultural patterns of food habits and dietary practices are fundamental in the maintenance

54

of health. If this is true, then a corresponding importance can be attached to the role of women in rural societies for two reasons. In the first place, they control the preparation of food for their families and are to a large extent the repository of 'food lore'. Second, their role includes everything connected with the birth of children and with care for them in infancy and in their early years, and it is in the early years that food habits are established.

The significance of culture patterns for nutrition workers

To introduce the concept of food patterns in a culture, use will be made of a table[1] (p. 56) intended to illustrate how social and cultural studies can be related to the preparation of nutrition workers in rural areas.

The divisions in the left-hand column represent, first, the cultural basis of a given society or community; second, the general food situation in terms of production and exchange; third, food consumption in the habitual family diets; and fourth, the nutritional condition of the general population and of the children. It is suggested that these four 'categories' of information are essential and inseparable in any nutritional survey or nutrition programme planning.

In the middle column these four main categories are broken up to relate the general situation to detailed investigations. The concept of patterns as suggested in this chapter is introduced in order that nutrition workers can realize that there can be an 'organizing frame' for assembling the details of ordinary living, which may otherwise be observed as a haphazard collection of customs. It is also intended to relate the consumption of food to the local internal market economy; to the fuel situation, especially where it is necessary to economize on fuel for cooking; to the demands of hospitality; and to the type of social organization which, at least in part, regulates the size and membership of cooking and eating groups. The right-hand column notes points arising from information derived from the middle column – points that should be emphasized in training health workers for rural work, or in planning programmes for discussion among groups of women in village meetings.

[1] Part of a background paper prepared by the writer for the Cuernavaca conference on Malnutrition and Food Habits (cf. Burgess and Dean, 1962), and used in a WHO/PAHO conference on how to apply social science concepts in the graduate training of health education workers.

TABLE I NUTRITIONAL STUDIES OF COMMUNITIES

Fields of knowledge	Social and economic factors involved in nutritional studies of communities	Implications of this study for training and teaching
I. The community and its culture	(a) The patterns of social grouping: family and kinship; status; work	The patterns of behaviour between groups and individuals
	(b) The pattern of adjustment to the environment	The patterns of authority in decision-making and in leadership
II. The food situation in general	(a) The use of local resources and the cultivation of foodstuffs	Attitudes to economic activities and to food production, both traditional and changing
	(b) The impact of local markets and of buying food at stores	Ideas about food and its functions
	(c) The ritual use of food at feasts and ceremonies	Changing fashions in foods
III. Family diets (habitual meals; snacks)	(a) Varying standards of living	Methods of household management
	(b) The balance between using and selling available foodstuffs	Intelligence and ability in house-wife's tasks
	(c) Fuel situation in relation to cooking	Time available for cooking, etc.
	(d) Type of family units making up cooking and eating groups	Social obligations of hospitality, food exchange, etc.
IV. Nutritional state of the population in general and of children under 5 years	(a) Composition of selected households – i.e. number of adults and children to be fed from household resources	Health teaching on nutrition: (a) general principles of adequate diets
	(b) The food of the children	(b) special needs of young children
	(c) The food of the adults, especially wage-earners and pregnant women	(c) meaning and signs of malnutrition

Emphasis on valuable elements in indigenous diets

So much is written in nutritional and diet studies about inadequate diets and malnutrition that some of the positive nutritional merits of indigenous diets as well as the element of pleasure in eating need attention. In contrast to the long list of 'taboos' which are often the *leit motif* of tropical nutrition studies, very few studies emphasize the esteem, often well founded scientifically, in which some local foods are held, or the pleasure in well-prepared food in general. It may be that campaigns to improve nutrition should begin by inviting attention to those elements in traditional food habits which are scientifically valuable as well as aesthetically pleasing to the consumers.

The 'world of knowledge' which rural people possess must not be underestimated (Tentori, 1962). The writer has noted the enthusiasm with which Ngoni children and young people pick and eat wild fruits, especially towards the end of the rains when their astringent properties are craved. The widespread use, again towards the end of the rains, of baobab and other fruits containing appreciable amounts of ascorbic acid has also been observed among the Gwembe Tonga. Although the greater importance of these fruits in the diet may be primarily a matter of taste, appearance, and relative abundance, it is not impossible that the Valley Tonga have somehow learned to emphasize those fruits which, nutritionally-speaking, are the best for them (Scudder, 1962, p. 209).

Some Eskimo (Lantis, 1959) make use of arctic willow and ground birch, both of which are known as sources of Vitamin C, and birch as a source of Vitamin B1 also. They dry and store fish eggs, eat birds' eggs fresh in their season, and prize seal-oil not merely as a food, but as the best single maintainer of good health. Similar traditional 'knowledge' is seen in the Somali cultural pattern of giving lightly cooked liver to pregnant women who show signs of anaemia, and extra milk during pregnancy and lactation.

The concept of the staple food

On the other hand, in most tropical areas the chief item of diet is a cooked cereal.

'The staple food, be it *matoke* or rice or some other cereal, seems to occupy a unique place in all the societies mentioned and is esteemed as *the* food, without which no one can get along. Other foods seem to be regarded more as flavoring than as health-giving agents in their own right. In fact, apart from the cereal staple, and the recognition of a connection between adequate feeding and strength, there seems to be less idea of foods having a positive effect on health, than of certain foods being harmful in certain circumstances. The adherence to the familiar staple, and the total lack of belief or satisfaction in the nourishing powers of any substitute has been demonstrated in times of famine and scarcity in India and elsewhere' (Burgess, 1960).

The rice-feeding ceremony in West Bengal is a traditional Hindu rite intended to emphasize the cultural importance of rice as a food. It occurs at the age of six months for a boy and seven months for a girl. The child is placed on his maternal uncle's knee, or his grandfather's, and fed boiled rice with some bitter or sour food, such as a sharp vegetable, curds, or buttermilk. Before the ceremony rice cannot be given to the child, and neither can *dal*, fish, or eggs. This does not mean that after the ceremony this total diet is introduced as a regular feature of child-feeding, mainly because curds and buttermilk are too expensive for daily use (Jelliffe, 1957, p. 130).

Cross-cultural confusions

The names given to foods often involve their properties, their preparation, and their effects on the body, so that the problems of understanding local terms are formidable because of the complicated traditional concepts that lie behind them. As an example, in one culture rice is a prestige food, desirable but not easily obtainable, and ideas about its use are built around this theme. In another it is 'the staff of life', the normal staple cereal diet; without it people have no strength to work, and it is therefore an absolute necessity. In yet another culture large rice meals are said to make people sleepy and mentally dull, and hence fit only for manual work, the implication here being that rice alone is not an adequate diet and that there should be beneficial and ample side dishes served with the rice. Questions to patients on what they know and think about rice or any other staple cereal in their normal diet have to be expressed in terms of the cultural background, for interpretation from one language to another can go far astray.

The idea of using fresh fish in the diet, where it is available but not eaten, and where protein intake is generally inadequate, will involve the questioner in an intricate maze of beliefs, expressed in local terminology about the properties of fresh fish, such as that it causes worms, that it is poisonous, that it induces impotence, and so on.

A study of the economy and of protein malnutrition among the Digo shows two examples of linguistic confusion arising from misinterpretation of terms and concepts. With regard to infant feeding:

'A woman should be able to devote considerable time to the rearing of her child during the first few years and she should be very careful in his diet. If she cannot provide sufficient milk of her own to feed the child, she may supplement this with cow, goat or tinned milk, or with a very thin gruel made from maize or cassava meal. . . . In most cases the only supplement to her own milk will be the gruel, both because the additional milk is expensive and because such gruel is believed to be completely adequate in itself, especially if fed in large quantities. A Digo will never give the infant other vegetables, fruits, meats, fish or eggs, either separately or as a relish for the gruel, for these are *chitoweo*. Only gruel, or *chakuria*, is a suitable substitute for mother's milk.

'Often western medical officials and community development workers in Digo country did not understand the difference between *chakuria* and *chitoweo*. To them, the African word for food of all types was the Swahili *chakula* similar to *chakuria*. African interpreters had become so accustomed to this terminology that they used it as well in translating the statements of Europeans who did not know enough Swahili. The unfortunate result was that western officials customarily advised Digo to feed their undernourished children more *chakula*. Digo could only reply that their children obtain more than enough *chakula*. Digo need to be told that their infants require *chitoweo*, for it is this which they do not get. They must be made aware that their *chakula* is not enough' (Gerlach, 1961).

Effects of food prejudices on health

People in all cultures, besides showing their preferences for certain kinds of food and certain ways of preparing them, show traditional prejudices against other foods, the reasons for which are in some cases lost in the past, in others very much alive today. In Yugoslavia, North Brazil, and Mexico recent attempts to introduce enriched corn or manioc meal were resisted by village women because they believe it could cause their men to become impotent. The same fear of becoming impotent lay behind the Ngoni men's refusal to eat greens or fresh fish.

In some countries there is a recent form of prejudice against eating hand-milled rice because polished rice from the mills is easier to handle and confers more prestige. A rigorous diet for pregnant women, prescribed by the senior women and indigenous practitioners in parts of rural Burma, consisting almost entirely of polished rice, led to increase in beriberi among the women and to acute infantile beriberi in breast-fed babies, causing many deaths (Sharma, 1955). Case studies of infantile and mother's beriberi showed family histories of infant deaths ranging from two out of three children up to eleven out of eleven. Scores of cases of infantile beriberi were successfully treated with massive doses of Vitamin B, orally and by injections to both mother and child. The infants thrive on breast-feeding as long as the mother continues with the prescribed diet, and never have to be treated again for vitamin deficiencies. The cultural component of food habits for pregnant women is illustrated in the fact that Chinese and Indian women living in the same Burmese rural villages do not lose children from breast-feeding as the poorer Burmese women do. The reasons are that as a diet for pregnant women the Indian women use parboiled rice and milk products, and the Chinese polished rice but taken with fish, meat, and eggs.

In many cultures the withdrawal of food is regarded as essential in the traditional treatment of childhood illnesses – particularly if diarrhoea is present. This may be fatal if the child is already undernourished. In Guatemala it was found that:

'The beliefs and practices regarding child feeding in a small rural Guatemalan Indian village contribute to the inadequacy of the diet. The concept of special food needs for the health of young children is almost non-existent. There is a strong tendency to avoid giving them foods of animal origin because these are thought to stimulate worms, and to withdraw protein-containing foods almost entirely when diarrhoea develops for any reason. For short term results it may be easier to introduce a new cereal product for the supplementary and mixed feeding of infants and young children than to overcome the prejudice surrounding milk, eggs, meat and similar foods. "Food" and "medicine" are completely distinct concepts in the culture, thus making it difficult to encourage the use of food to regain or promote health' (Solien and Scrimshaw, 1957).

Malnutrition in preschool children

Nutrition and paediatric studies at the present time are showing clearly the results of malnutrition in children aged 1–4. Some of the factors in child malnutrition which emerge from the studies in many parts of the world are:

1. There is no doubt that the primary cause of inadequate children's diets lies in the economic level of the families. Obtaining enough food and the right food for all members of the family is beyond the reach of the poorest classes in all societies.

2. The second basic factor is the absence of elementary knowledge, or even awareness, of the relation between food intake and health, and between food and physical development. The culture patterns of beliefs about food show a general absence of knowledge of this relationship, which vitally affects the health and growth of children.

3. The third factor, which follows on from this, is that the cultural practice of reliance on their customary staple food leads people to believe that it is also the best food for children, who are regarded in so many societies as 'little adults', and since they are smaller than grown-ups, therefore they need less food or a diluted form of the staple cereal.

4. The fourth factor, the 'order at meals', is also a deeply embedded cultural practice. The men who are the productive members of the family have the first choice at meals and the largest share of the food prepared. The mother and the small children come last in the process of being served portions of the food.

5. The fifth factor is the long gap between meals that occurs when mothers have to work away from home. At the evening meal children cannot eat enough of the bulky cereal to meet their needs. Their hunger is sometimes temporarily appeased in cultural situations where cooked food is sold in villages or on the roadside and children beg for money to buy 'snacks'. But such a practice does not provide the balanced meals the small child needs for healthy growth.

THE ROLE OF WOMEN RELATED TO
HEALTH PRACTICES AND PROBLEMS

In attempting to analyse cultural patterns in relation to people's attitudes and practices towards health and sickness, it becomes clear that studies cannot get far without intensive investigation of women's role in their society. This is a field beset by misleading generalizations about women's 'low status', generalizations that are often made without adequate examination of a woman's responsibilities in her different spheres. This is particularly true in tropical rural societies where women have so much to do outside as well as inside their homes.

The following guide-lines are suggested to relate woman's role in tropical rural societies to health practices and problems: first, her inter-personal marriage and kinship relations; next, her activities in her home; then outside her home; and finally, the sociological setting of childbirth practices.

Relations with husband and with kinship group

Of a woman's personal relationships in her marriage the dominant one is that of sexual partner to her husband. Unless she can satisfy and please him in this regard, he can probably divorce her – he will cer-tainly ignore her. She therefore wants to stimulate and retain his desire for her, while observing the required avoidance of intercourse during menstruation, and at culturally determined periods before and after childbirth. Where the women are insecure, economically or socially, as in some Moslem cultures, they dread divorce and therefore they place a high value on their husband's approval. This may lead them to cook only the familiar dishes which they know will please, and discourage attempts at trying out newer and more nourishing foods. In a poly-gamous society a wife may be competing for her husband with other wives, and her relationship with her co-wives will be a role she has to learn, and to watch continuously. If she goes to live in her husband's village on marriage, either in a joint family household or in some less closely circumscribed residential group, her role as daughter-in-law towards her mother-in-law will again be a matter of constant adjust-ment and attention. In Ngoni society, girls are taught before marriage what this process of adjustment will involve. They can indeed see it with their own eyes in the behaviour of young wives in the village who come as strangers to their husbands' families. The Ngoni marriage songs are full of the grief and tension that the young bride must feel on leaving the relative freedom of her father's home when she marries. Yet all her previous teaching leads up to that moment, instructing her how she must identify herself with her husband's people, produce children for his family, and contribute to the integrity and stability of the new family group which she has joined on marriage.

Relations with children

Finally, a woman has her relations with her own children, particularly close with the latest baby, less intimate with the ex-baby and older children. Again, her relations with the children follow a cultural pattern, ranging from one in which she has virtually no say about how to rear them, especially in relation to their food and health, to one where the modern influence of education and perhaps a degree of economic independence bring about some determination on the part of the mother to carry out new ideas.

Activities within the home

Within her home, unless she is sharing the household of a joint family and her work is allotted to her, it is her responsibility to sweep and keep clean the premises, prepare and cook the food, and organize its distribution at meal-times. The Ngoni regard very highly this role of the 'divider' – *mgawira* – he or she who divides out the available cooked food from one cooking pot to the eating dishes allotted to adults and children. At big feasts the men divide the meat and the women the cereals and vegetables and groundnut sauces. The women also divide out the highly prized cooked blood of a recently killed beast, and the milk curds brought to them by the herd boys. A woman's reputation for common sense and justice often stems from her proven ability to 'divide' food equitably according to the cultural pattern.

The importance of this role as the divider of food, and the way in which it is carried out, are not unrelated to more general skills in home management. The quality of being 'house-proud' is widely esteemed by women who live in very simple surroundings, and they display it when they have a sense of order and keep their house and its rudimentary equipment clean and shining. These are obviously important qualities for health workers to look out for when talking with village women about hygiene in the home.

It is in the home, or on the veranda in the sun, that a woman nurses a sick child or sick husband or relative. The kind of care exercised, the food and drink given or withheld, and the precautions taken are laid down in the training of the woman and are part of the traditional culture of her society.

F

63

Activities outside the home

Outside the home a village woman has the daily task of fetching water for all household needs. She may take clothes to be washed near the source of the water supply – spring, stream, canal, or well. But she has to carry and store all water for herself and her family for drinking, cooking, washing pots and pans, and washing the baby and younger children. Fuel is a constant problem for the rural housewife. Village women may have to devote the greater part of a day to fetching fuel, or to making and drying fuel cakes from cattle dung; and in dry weather they may have to go for their water any distance from a short walk of 200 yards to one of two or three or more miles.

In many village areas women share in, or carry, the main burden of cultivation of the cereal crop except for the heavy initial work of clear-ing and preparing the land. In a yam-growing area of East Nigeria, cassava was introduced as a crop that could withstand locusts and drought. The women took up cassava cultivation enthusiastically, leaving the yams as the traditional men's crop. This gave the women more work to do, but it brought them a measure of economic inde-pendence. A study made of this situation (Ottenberg, 1959) shows that the women who sell cassava flour in the markets are now interested in better standards of living, better nutrition, and in education for their children. Ironically, it is the nutritionally poorer food crop, which the men despise, that gives the needed impetus to the women to stand on their own feet and look ahead. Women not only do a large share of the cultivation in many rural areas, particularly the arduous and backbreak-ing task of transplanting rice, but, when the crops begin to ripen, they and their small children may have to live in huts on the fields, scaring away birds, baboons, and other marauders, thus exposing themselves to additional hazards, as we have seen.

Systems of marketing and trading carried on by women as an integral part of their cultural role have given women in some societies a high degree of economic independence, though not always or necessarily associated with an interest in improving general standards of living, and especially of health and nutrition.

In Togoland the roles of rural women show wide cultural variations:

'The status of women, including the relations between men and women and the extent and nature of the influence they could exercise on each other, varied within the region, affected by kinship structure, economic activities, and in some areas (with one woman, one vote) political considerations. A young Konkomba woman, assimilated into her husband's lineage and dominated by her husband's mother was in a very different position, and had different values and interests, from the prosperous market woman of a matrilineal area. There were many varieties of non-kinship association, ranging from the little group fetching water together and visiting each other's houses to highly organized religious, political and market associations' (Spens, 1960).

Implications for health workers

Two conclusions emerge from a survey of some recorded studies and reports on the role a woman has to perform in village and rural life, a daily routine varied only by seasonal occupations and occasional extra claims from a sick person in the family. One concerns the problem of time in a woman's day. This emerges in several reports about their unwillingness or apparent inability to attend at clinics, either for treatment for themselves or with a sick or well baby. Such a visit may well take up half a day or the best part of a day, and throw out of gear all the woman's necessary daily routine. The timing of this daily routine can perhaps be planned more efficiently so as to give the women some leisure, and it is evident that the provision of more village amenities, such as a nearby water supply or a corn mill, eases the burden of the routine. More leisure can affect the women's readiness not only to go to clinics but among other things to do more 'mothering' of their children. Certain studies of child health have emphasized the lack of mothering, particularly for the ex-baby, who so often falls victim to *kwashiorkor*. A rapid and more lasting recovery from *kwashiorkor* has been found to occur in those children who have good mothering while in hospital and on their return home (Géber and Dean, 1956).

Since this question of time in a woman's day is so closely connected with her role as wife, mother, and 'provider', it is important that the health worker should not regard the problem only from her own point of view as an educated town-dweller, looking at conditions in village homes from an external superficial angle. This leads on to the next conclusion: that there is a great need for more studies of rural women's life, carried out *in situ* in a village setting. The cultural implications of the way a society is organized in its social and economic life, and also the cultural changes taking place in that society – changes due to improved transport, better water supplies, fencing of vegetable gardens, organization of women's clubs, and so on – need to be analysed.

Traditional birth practices

A universal aspect of women's role in rural life is their association with the conduct of childbirth. Many brief reports and other longer studies have been made by nurses and doctors of birth practices in traditional cultures, and most anthropologists include some reference to the subject when dealing with social groups and social behaviour. It is not as a rule difficult therefore for health workers to find out and put together the details of actual birth practices, as well as the kinds of advice and regulations laid down in the cultural pattern for a pregnant woman and for her conduct after the birth has taken place.

The importance of this kind of knowledge for public health programmes and health workers is twofold. In the first place it is on these traditional lines that the vast majority of births take place in rural areas in tropical countries. This is the sphere in which women have most power and authority, and those wielding much of this authority are the older women, tradition-oriented for the most part. There are cultural areas, as in parts of Nigeria and Ghana, where the women, and the community at large, accept with enthusiasm the help of trained midwives with their new, hygienic, and skilled methods of conducting labour and caring for the mother and child after the birth. An interest in modern birth practices is not always, however, allied with scientific views on the nutrition of the mother when pregnant or lactating.

This opens up the second reason why knowledge of traditional birth practices and of the attitudes and beliefs inherent in them is of importance. The training of local traditional birth attendants, and of younger women who want to take training in midwifery, has to be related to this field of knowledge at every stage. And the field of knowledge cannot be encompassed by an enumeration of what actually takes place when the woman calls the midwife and the baby is born.

It is useful to make some distinction between the two kinds of help available to a woman in childbirth, which are inherent in the traditional culture. In the first instance, a woman will get help from a small group of relatives and friends. In the second, a group may be present, but the actual delivery will be performed by a traditional birth attendant who may or may not be a member of the kin group of the woman or her husband.

66

The role of the group who assist the woman is partly psychological – to encourage the woman during labour. They may sit round her in the house, or just outside, and chant little songs with a refrain such as: 'Sheep have children, and they have no pain. You will have no pain when your child is born.' In some cultures the woman is looked after by her mother and her maternal relatives, often going to her mother's home for the birth, especially of the first child. In cultures where the patrilineal principle is dominant, the woman is attended by her husband's mother and his relatives, because the new child will be part of his family. Since the woman in labour is in this latter case more or less a stranger to the family, the women who conduct the birth are inclined to be stern and unsympathetic towards her. She on her part dare not utter a cry or show any evidence of pain, lest her own family and her upbringing should be disgraced by her conduct.

In many parts of Latin America, some Islamic countries, India, and parts of South-East Asia, there are women in both rural and urban areas who are traditional birth attendants; a linguistic term denotes their office, which has a recognized significance in relation to their role and their status in the society.

A recent study was carried out in Mexico (de Sandoval, 1963) on the work and practices of the empirical midwife, known as *partera empirica* or *comadrona*. The objective was to provide information that might be used in training courses. Although this study was made in an urban setting, it was in an economically depressed community, and its findings include several points that are of general significance. In the first place a large majority of the empirical midwives interviewed (87·4 per cent), though they had all lived ten years in Mexico City, had begun their work in their own home towns. The main reason why a particular *comadrona* is engaged by a woman is that either she or her mother has attended the woman's mother in a rural town. Thus there are ties other than those of propinquity or alleged skill between the calling of a particular *comadrona* and the woman she is to help; and there is an established confidence based on experience.

Another interesting finding is that the services of the *comadrona* begin long before the birth, even though the woman may also attend a prenatal clinic:

'One important fact that emerged from the study was that 92·5 per cent of the "midwives" give pre-natal guidance to their clients – in the form of instructions which may vary very considerably. This means that they consider it important for the women to receive advice in this period, although the advice they give is based on their traditional ideas and prejudices, so that in many cases they succeed in frightening the pregnant woman and also in making themselves indispensable; they demand blind obedience on the part of their clients and insist that they must "consult" them at regular intervals. In many cases, the woman is accompanied by her husband who takes the occasion to arrange for the "midwife" to attend the birth, and to agree upon the fee. The "midwife" also acts as adviser on matrimonial matters and family difficulties; as a rule she looks after the children when they are ill, especially in the first year, and advises on the food to be given to the infant – who thus becomes the victim of the ignorance of the mother and of the "midwife".'

The third point arising out of the study is the prestige of the *comadrona*. This is of particular interest because they have no legal recognition of any kind, and are in fact pursuing their activities outside the law – a situation that made getting some of the information very difficult. In spite of the difficulties inherent in their occupation, it was found that 93·56 per cent of the *comadrona* are very satisfied with the prestige they enjoy. Many of them baptize the children at the request of the parents, and are consulted by the community when adults and children are sick.

An earlier study made in Peru (Wellin, 1953) posed three leading questions of wide general importance, although related to descriptions of the local birth practices. The first was: what are the beliefs, action-patterns, and techniques, and to what broader cultural values do they belong? The second: what are the interpersonal relationships, and how do the people involved interact with one another? The third: what are the emotional attitudes, including the pleasantly toned emotions as well as the fears and anxieties?

Many of the points occurring in the Mexican study reflect on one or more of these questions, and are further illustrated in the Peru study. For example, the role of the *partera* in Peru confers very little status in urban society but a high one in rural areas. This status is partly related to her knowledge, not only of delivery and postnatal care but also of cultural ideas about food, 'hot' and 'cold' ideology, and how to use herbal remedies. It is also connected with her age, her experience as mother, grandmother, and *partera*, and her local residence and long connexion with the area where she is known and trusted, and has served the same group of families.

This comfort-conferring relationship arising from the services of the *partera*, and from the customary presence of the husband at the home delivery, is contrasted strongly with confinement at a hospital. In difficult or abnormal labour, hospital treatment is recommended by the *partera* and appreciated by the woman patient. But in relatively normal conditions, for most rural women, hospital confinement appears to be a fear-producing, anxiety-ridden situation. This is in part an outcome of the impersonal, commanding attitudes of hospital personnel, who set up a social and cultural gulf between themselves and their patients by addressing them in the second person singular, as if they were children. Hospital régimes in food and washing strike discordant and unpleasant notes for the rural women, who are apprehensive about the treatment of the baby, and especially about the fact that so many people are 'seeing' or 'eyeing' the child, whom they may not have been able to protect with the customary red ribbon to ward off the evil eye.

A deep-rooted practice in many cultures when deliveries are in the home is to keep the woman and baby in seclusion in the place of birth for a stated period after childbirth. The period of seclusion may vary from ten to forty days and may be accompanied by prohibitions about cooking, about the eating of certain kinds of food, and about who is permitted to come in and see the mother and baby. Her helpers recognize the need for the mother to rest, and, in the case of her firstborn, to learn how to handle and feed the baby. They, or the local birth attendant, also advise her on how to promote lactation which, in societies where the economic level is low, is a source of great anxiety for the woman until it is well established.

The underlying reason for the period of seclusion is, in very many societies, the fear of pollution from the woman who has given birth. The ceremony known as 'coming out of the house' at the end of the seclusion period is always preceded by a ritual bath for the woman and child, and a thorough (in a ritual and hygienic sense) cleaning of the house and everything that was in it at the time of birth that had not been previously burned. The ritual bath is separate in intention from the preliminary washing of the mother and child immediately after delivery, which is sometimes followed by no further washing until the period of seclusion is over.

CHAPTER 7

Ritual, religion, and values in health practices

A ritual practice affects a health campaign

In several reports of malaria-eradication campaigns references occur to people's actions in and reactions to spraying operations. A special study of these reactions was carried out by the Central Health Education Burea in India among tribal groups in Orissa (Dhillon and Karm, 1961). The people in the villages investigated showed that they are aware that the incidence of malaria has declined, but they do not associate this with spraying operations, which they nevertheless submit to, allegedly for fear of prosecution. Those in charge of the campaign found that to some considerable extent the spraying is made less effective as a deterrent, owing to the cultural practice of frequent plastering of the houses, both inside and out. This is mainly a ritual plastering carried out on an average eight to ten times a year to celebrate festivals; to remove pollution after a death, or childbirth, or a recovery from smallpox; and to prepare for a marriage. In addition to these established ritual occasions, the housewife replasters the house whenever she wants it to look nice.

RITUAL AND THE HEALING PROCESS

All societies, everywhere, have forms of ritual which are built into their culture and performed with traditional ceremony. Most rituals are group activities, or are performed by an individual on behalf of the welfare of a group, as in the case of the housewife plastering the house. They consist of formalized actions, sometimes associated with a traditional form of words, and they may or may not have easily perceptible religious or magical significance. Nevertheless, in many cultures the performance of ritual is connected with religious beliefs about the relationship of human beings to the supernatural forces in the universe. We have seen how this idea is fundamental in the Navaho performance of the healing ritual, which in restoring a sick person to health aims at restoring harmony or equilibrium between the patient, his kin group, and the spiritual universe. Studies of indigenous systems of medicine in India bring out the same deeply felt need for a restoration of harmony with unseen forces. Sickness is regarded by the village people as a moral as well as a physical crisis, involving human conduct and cosmic purpose. For example, for a person suffering from physical weakness due to malnutrition and anaemia the western medical cure is to prescribe an iron tonic and vitamins. The Hindu cure is to prescribe a ritual pilgrimage to a holy place involving ritual baths (Carstairs, 1955).

The examples of the Navaho healing ritual and of the Hindu ritual pilgrimage emphasize the gulf in thinking and concepts between the western scientific approach to health (based on a cultural acceptance of scientific principles and allowing for some distinction between secular and sacred spheres of thought and action) and the widespread denial of such a concept of culture in much of the rest of the world.

RELIGIOUS IDEOLOGY UNDERLYING HEALTH PRACTICES

A series of articles in the *Health Education Journal* (Vol. 17, 1959) surveyed the influence of several of the world's great religions on health education among their members. The articles, contributed by medical personnel who were nationals of the countries concerned, referred chiefly to rules about personal and public hygiene enforced by religious sanctions, and to prescribed rules about abstinence and restrictions in regard to food and water on given occasions determined, in special circumstances, by religious observance. The authors considered that if the practices enjoined were strictly observed many of them contributed to personal and public wellbeing. A religious ideology underlying health practices not only codifies health behaviour but gives an additional sense of security to those who adhere to the precepts.

One of the major components of a people's culture is the complex of their beliefs about the relation of man to nature, of man to his fellowmen, and of man to those supernatural powers which he recognizes as controlling the universe. These beliefs are incorporated in their cosmology, their philosophy, and their religion. Their understanding about life and death, health, illness, and accidents is embedded in this complex. Widespread in many religious systems is the concept that illness and premature death are a punishment for infringing an ethical code or failing to observe religious requirements. The Ngoni believed that when a warrior was wounded in battle his wounds would not heal unless his wife at home was observing strict sexual abstinence. References have already been made to the concept that the parents' infringement of the sexual code could cause *kwashiorkor* in a child. Medical psychiatrists treating mental health symptoms detect the extreme neurotic anxiety arising from a consciousness of having ignored a sexual code.

RITUAL IN RELATION TO ILLNESS, BIRTH, AND DEATH

The place of ritual in the complex of beliefs about the origin and incidence of illness is largely protective – to prevent the occurrence of illness – but it is also an act of purification and of healing. The exorcism of evil spirits, the observance of taboos, the votive offering to allay anxiety, the reintegration of a group after the death of one of its members – these are all ritual acts and occasions related to cultural beliefs about life and the supernatural.

In most cultures pregnancy and birth are not associated with illness, but they are regarded as a 'dangerous period' during which the woman and the new-born child are exposed to many perils which must be guarded against by traditional ritual. Nor is the element of danger present only for the woman and her child, since, as we saw in the last chapter, ritual precautions are often taken to safeguard the rest of the family from the danger of pollution associated with the process of birth.

Death also is frequently associated with pollution. In some cultures those who handle and bury the corpse are thought to be polluted. In others a bereaved person, especially a widow, is feared for her potentially evil effect on the health of the rest of the family, because it is thought that she may be in some way associated with the cause of death of her husband. In certain African matrilineal societies, the husband is held to account for his wife's death, and the ritual of 'taking the death off him' has to be performed before he can be considered 'safe' to associate with any other woman.

Mourning rituals

Many of the forms of mourning ritual are designed to remove pollution and to bring together and to reintegrate the living group that has lost one of its members, and, if possible, to protect them all from future ills. Among some African peoples not only is the living group of kin brought together for the successive stages of the mourning ritual but the 'gap' that has been caused by death is closed through filling the relationships left vacant by the death. Among the Malawi Cewa, for example, the mother's brother plays an all-important role in the guardianship of his sister's children. If he should die, someone has to 'enter into his place' and take over the role and responsibilities of a maternal uncle. This is sometimes called 'successional inheritance', and the change in name as well as in the relationship and functions of the individuals concerned can bewilder those unfamiliar with the culture. Another form of closing the gap after death is connected with the ancestor cult, when (as among the Ngoni) the spirit of an important dead person is 'brought back' to his village after a mourning period, and is 'placed under the guardianship' of a senior woman who takes care of the ritual vessels associated with sacrifices to the ancestors.

In one Central American area, when a child dies in hospital the parents cannot bear to have their child buried by the hospital. They want to take the body home, dress it in the child's best clothes, and bury it in a cemetery where they can go and visit the grave. In this way only can they carry out the ritual that will respect the dead and integrate the living with his memory. In some Islamic countries it is believed that an 'innocent' child who dies will support the parents in Paradise. Much the same belief is found in parts of Latin America, where the dead child is thought to become a little angel able to help the family left on earth. Here again the chief concept behind the ritual of mourning is that of continued association of the dead with the family.

OBLIGATION ON GROUP TO PARTICIPATE

Rituals connected with fertility and birth, and those connected with the threat of severe illness, and with death, burial, and mourning, illustrate how human mating and fertility, the birth of a child, the illness or death of a member of a family, are concerns of a group of people, not of one or two individuals. The obligation to take part in the appropriate ritual is binding on all the members of the group. In Ngoni villages when a death occurred and some members of the kin group could not be present at the time of the burial, they were obliged to go through an abbreviated form of the ritual of mourning before they either slept or ate food in the houses of their relatives. The writer saw several young men on their return to their village from working at a distance go through this ritual of respect for the dead and reintegration with the living before they settled down to the welcome prepared for them by their relatives.

The role of fear

A study of the rituals of kinship among the Nyakyusa in Tanganyika describes how fear of *not* partaking in the ritual is related to the overriding importance of social relationships:

> 'The rituals express the fear and teach men what they must do to be saved. They teach them to cooperate with their kinsmen and to follow traditional custom, for in that alone does salvation lie. The fear of madness or of sterility compels each generation to follow traditional custom as ordained for them by the heroes: thus is the dependence of man upon his society instilled. . . . It is no accident that the Nyakyusa interpret all the rituals, and especially the death ritual, as a protection against going mad, against the disintegration of the personality. And safety is assured to the living by following minutely the traditions of their lineage' (Wilson, 1957, p. 232).

The author goes on to say that the nature of these fears is culturally determined, and that 'the rituals do not create fear out of nothing. All the situations in which they are performed – birth and death, marriage and misfortune – are situations of emotional tension in all societies. The rituals heighten the emotions and canalise them.'

The earlier passage quoted refers to the fear of sterility in a family or lineage if ritual requirements are not carried out in minute detail. There is evidence in many areas of a widespread fear of sterility, which sends many women to make votive offerings and to carry out other rituals to avert or to remove the stigma of sterility and to induce conception. This accounts for the association in many cultures of female puberty rituals with the fertility of humans and of crops. In a certain Cewa village in Malawi it was obligatory for the headman of the village, the senior male member of the matrilineal lineage, to abstain from all sexual intercourse during the prolonged puberty rites for nubile girls, and during the ritual performed for a married woman's first pregnancy. On one occasion a series of misfortunes that occurred, including food shortages, were attributed to the negligence of the headman to observe these ritual taboos.

However obscure the meaning of some of the rituals connected with life and death may be to people outside a particular culture, to those

74

inside the culture the actions and words of the ritual and their participation in it have a profound significance:

'Men express in ritual what moves them most: the form of expression is conventional and obligatory, and therefore in ritual the values of a group (as opposed to those of individuals) are revealed. Treating food, and reproduction, and family relationships and the community as sacred, expresses the importance of these things to the group concerned, and at the same time breeds respect for them. Treating them as important in ritual makes people feel that they are important' (Wilson, 1957, p. 229).

BELIEF IN THE PROTECTIVE FUNCTION OF RITUAL

Implications for modern preventive medicine programmes
Health personnel who advocate preventive health measures should realize that much of the traditional ritual in a culture appears to the people concerned as a form of protection for individuals and for human groups. It is a kind of preventive action supported by traditional beliefs about the causes of illness. It is often more than this, for positive health may be closely connected in people's thinking with the punctilious observance of rituals, and, conversely, illness may result from non-observance. The fear of madness, the fear of sterility, the fear of pollution are haunting fears. Some understanding of the protective nature of the ritual performed is vital to the success of introducing preventive medicine programmes to communities with a different concept of prevention.

'The war between good and evil'
In societies that have an ancestor cult the spirits of ancestors are usually regarded as playing an ambivalent role. Ancestors of a person's own lineage or clan may be regarded as generally benevolent, but prone to show disapproval of incorrect or antisocial behaviour on the part of their descendants by causing illness or failure of crops. On the other hand, ancestral spirits of another clan than one's own, with whom in the past there may have been overt or latent hostility, may show this hostility by striking at the descendants of their former enemies. 'The war between good and evil is always going on' is a fundamental concept shared by many societies, and it has as a sequel the concept that good

75

life, good health, and good luck proceed in an unbroken line if not disturbed by evil influences. People look around for explanations of disasters in the physical and the human world, and through the systems of divination responsibility is fixed on some living person or some dead ancestor, or some other malicious spirit.

The prevailing fear of the evil eye in so many societies illustrates this sense of human malice lurking near and the need for protection against it. A healthy child is not safe from the jealousy of other women, and the mother of the child fears the effects of this human jealousy and the possible evil magical forces which can operate through it and harm her child. So she does her best to conceal the child's health and good looks by dressing it in dirty clothes, giving it a false name, or a girl's name if it is a boy.

Traditional avoidances and preventive actions

In the midst of known and unknown menaces, people seek for a refuge and an escape. To begin with they take such preventive action for themselves and their children as is sanctioned by their cultural pattern and accepted as a means of warding off disaster. They observe taboos of many kinds. Menstruating women, for example, are prohibited from many activities, including in some societies putting salt into the food they are cooking, lest they bring illness on their husband and children. People adhere rigidly to dietary rules which are believed to prevent specific illness or general conditions of ill health, such as the food regulations for pregnant women and for young children. One of the preventive actions very commonly followed is the constant recourse to laxatives, purgatives, and emetics. This may be to ward off or get rid of the possible effects of sorcery, if it is thought that the charms worn against sorcery are not powerful enough. It may be, however, that the local concept of health involves keeping the body system clear, and, as among the Samburu in Kenya, there may be a strong belief that all disease is a kind of poison which gets into the body and can be expelled only by purgatives made from medicinal plants.

People acquire a certain sense of confidence in following traditionally prescribed actions which are alleged to confer immunity against possible disaster. Among these is the wearing of amulets by children and adults. A nurse in East Pakistan observed that wearing amulets is a source of great comfort, and that they are 'handled lovingly in times of stress'. The continued use of amulets among the Digo illustrates the belief in their efficacy, since, if the parents break sexual taboos and the children do not suffer from *kwashiorkor*, then they conclude that the amulets worn by parents and children are effective.

Among the Swahili coastal villages in Kenya there is an annual ceremony of communal exorcism. At the beginning of each cultivating year when the rains are over, a cow is led round the village, readings of the Koran are held, and the cow is killed and eaten. The significance of this ritual act is to offer a sacrifice to God to keep away disease and to drive away evil spirits which could possess a person or a family.

The new shrines in Ghana serve those seeking protection from possible future evils and evildoers:

'Mentally ill people comprise only a very small proportion of the pilgrims who flock to these shrines not only from within Ashanti but from distant parts of Akan Ghana. The great majority are healthy people supplicating for "protection". Financially successful men are full of fear lest envious kinsmen should, by means of bad magic or witchcraft, bring about their ruin. Unsuccessful men are convinced that envious malice is the cause of their failure. . . . The typical pilgrim comes annually to the shrine, asks the deity for a year's protection and promises a thank offering of a sheep and a bottle of rum at the end of the year. The deity's protection and blessing is granted conditionally on the supplicant's keeping prescribed rules of ethical conduct' (Field, 1960, p. 37).

INFLUENCE OF CULTURAL VALUES ON HEALTH

The kind of protection that people seek through the performance of ritual suggests a deeper layer of thought and attitude behind ceremonies, acts, and forms of words. Values, and people's value systems, are elusive and intangible elements in a culture, but nevertheless exert a potent and enduring influence on their way of living. They are also the ultimate clue to people's response to health and welfare programmes, and to the acceptance of new practices in diet, child care, environmental hygiene, and so on.

'If planners are baffled about the non-acceptance of a program, they say "We must look for people's values about so and so. That will tell us what incentives to use." Incentives and values do not lie around on the surface of village life like dry maize stalks on the ground.

77

The anthropologist has good reason for appearing to stall, if he is suddenly asked to suggest what incentives could be used to persuade people to boil the water or to use a latrine or to give young children eggs to eat. Frequently public health planners are aware that if they want to get off to a good start, they should build on the villagers' preferences for certain improvements in daily living – that is for certain amenities such as a near-by water supply. . . . Planners, however, often do not know how to discover these preferences, nor how to rate them in terms of priorities. Still less are they able to explain to themselves or the public health personnel working in the area why there is local resistance to a program, and to relate this resistance to the fact that the villagers apparently set a very high value on retaining a particular practice.

'There is no short cut to the understanding by an outsider of the particular aspects of a prohibition or a practice which is tenaciously held by a group of people. Even when village people have grasped intellectually that a particular practice has no scientific validity, or even that it is dangerous to health, they may still adhere to it because they respect the authority of the older women who insist on it; or because giving it up might anger the ancestors who in turn might "trouble" the village; or because it had ritual connections with other practices, and could not be discarded without throwing doubt on a whole range of attitudes and practices instilled at puberty, marriage or pregnancy ceremonies' (Read, 1957, pp. 20–21).

Cross-cultural identification of values

The difficulties of understanding the basic values of a culture or sub-culture other than our own are not insuperable, though they are formidable. Anthropologists who could give a lead here are frequently not available or near at hand; and even if they are, they may not be interested in problems of health, or in elucidating people's attitudes to sickness and to modern medicine in terms of the problems put to them by health workers. If social science guidance is not immediately available, health personnel have to rely on their own resources, with such help in understanding the place of values in a people's culture as this and similar books have given them. There are two approaches on which health personnel might focus in their search for the values that neither sick nor well people readily talk about, although they in fact colour all their attitudes.

Values underlying ritual and religious ceremonies

One approach is to try to discover the occasions on which cultural values are stressed and made articulate. Some of these occasions are when certain kinds of ritual are carried out. Religious ceremonies emphasize, to those who participate in them, their concepts about the nature of the universe, how the supernatural elements in the universe impinge on man in his life on earth, and how this concept in turn affects the relation of man to his fellow-men. Deep in the complex of these beliefs is a concept that man can do little by himself to achieve health and wellbeing, and hence he places high in his scale of values all ceremonies and practices that maintain and restore balance and harmony between human beings and the supernatural. Among the Navaho:

'Maintaining health is one of the foci of traditional Navaho values. . . . Health is the central objective in religious behavior and represents the correct balance between man and his total physical, social and supernatural environment. Virtually all Navaho religious acts and ceremonies are focussed on a patient; the central endeavor is to drive out "evil" as it is manifested by disease and to welcome goodness and health' (Adair, 1958).

Values attached to food and its uses

Occasions on which values, or a particular value, are evident are not confined to ritual or to religious ceremonies. Handling the ordinary material things of life may express a deeply felt value. An Egyptian physician wrote[1] that bread had always been associated with worship of the gods. In the Pharaohic days it was carried to the temples and offered to the priests and gods. This attitude to handling bread is part of the lesson Egyptian children in rural areas learn early in life:

'Bread is not only filling, but also possesses an aura of sacredness, being believed to be the essence of life. The name given to bread is *aish* which literally means life. It is profane to put bread on the ground, and every effort must be made to pick up any crumb that falls to the ground for fear of it being trodden on. . . . Children are also enjoined to kiss bread if it falls from their hands on the ground, and if they find it lying in the street to remove it into a crevice in the wall' (Ammar, 1954, p. 34).

[1] Personal communication.

In the category of values attached to food and its uses are the concepts of 'hot' and 'cold' foods, their effects on health and sickness, the dangers inherent in not observing these qualities, and their interaction on disease when giving food to children and sick people.

Water, as in sacred rivers like the Ganges and the Nile, can enshrine cherished values. In a study of bilharziasis in Egypt, two physicians (Abdou and Omran, n.d.) spoke of the popular prevailing value attached to the Nile water, ever-flowing and everlasting, good for the fertility of the land and of human beings. Conversely, so they reported, pure drinking water from underground sources is held to bestow no blessing, and is even believed to undermine sexual powers.

The transmission of cultural values

The second approach to studies of values is suggested by the fact that cultural values in any society have to be learned. This means that children and young people in the process of growing up have to be taught how to behave to people, and how to handle the materials of livelihood, so that they may observe and respect, and not violate, the value system of their family and society. The objective of this training is so to guide and control children that they will become 'good adults' – capable of adjusting to the demands of the society to which they belong.

In order to reach the standards of adult behaviour which incorporate and respect cultural values, part of the child-training in many societies consists in letting children observe, imitate, and assist adults in the general conduct of domestic living. For example, in the course of child-training in an Egyptian village:

'The villagers express the educational process through emphasizing life and time as the most important educational agencies which mold and influence the character, and provide the experience. The difference between an adult and a child is, on the whole, quantitative rather than qualitative. The former knows and thus conforms to the cultural norms, while the latter does not. . . .

'The process of growing up is envisaged as a way of disciplining the child to conform to the adults' standards, and to comply with what their elders expect them to do, thus acquiring the qualities of being polite – "muaddab". . . . To become "muaddab" is the ideal set up by parents for their children, and the adherence to which is constantly impressed upon them.

'The word "muaddab" is applied to a child who defecates outside the house at the age of three or four, and goes further and further away from the house as he grows older. . . . A boy is "muaddab" if he recognizes that he should sit in the back row on going to the mosque. . . .

'The ideal norm of "adab" is a value which also has its religious sanction, as a pious son (ibn salih) is synonymous with "muaddab". Such a value does not only include the child's economic services and his observance of the expected social behavior, but also implies a pattern of reciprocity between child and family. A father who neglects the care of his "polite" children may be frequently exposed to illness, failure of crop, or death of cattle. Moreover, a family that infringes on the moral and religious code may consequently have sickly children' (Ammar, 1954, p. 125).

Close observation by the writer of life in Ngoni families and villages brought out not only the cultural values impressed on children but also on what occasions and by which methods such values are taught. Among these methods is the reiterated use of proverbs, often with a hidden meaning which children have to think about. At every meal-time behavioural values are emphasized, not only how to eat neatly with the fingers, but to avoid snatching greedily at food, especially at food which is in scarce supply and highly prized, like beef and chicken, to masticate quietly, and to rinse the mouth and use a twig toothbrush after each meal. In the same way, when anyone in a household is ill, the care of the sick person, the kinds of remark made about the possible cause of illness, and the decisions about treatment, all form learning situations for children and young people about values and beliefs in sickness. Their reiteration and visual reality are far more impressive than hygiene lessons taught from a book in school. The Ngoni have a well-integrated system of values in which respect for the ancestors, good behaviour to senior people, self-control in times of hunger, anger, and physical danger are all related to the maintenance of good health (Read, 1960).

Another observer describes the instruction of young people about the natural world in which they live and on which their food and health depend. Eskimo values are related to the harsh nature of their environment and their former total dependence on it for their livelihood. This cultural value gives the Eskimo a profound respect for animal life as well as for that of his fellow-men:

81

'The Eskimo did not under-estimate any creature: each has its own power which may affect man. Conservation, then, meant returning the sea animal's spirit to the ocean so it could be reborn and return to the place where it had received proper ritualistic treatment. Besides conserving life, what he considered the essential part of life, man turned to the sources of life. This meant a journey by the shaman's spirit to the deity protecting sea mammals or other animals to make sure this protector would send the animals to hungry human beings' (Lantis, 1957).

Since the natural world offers many hazards to life, young people are given knowledge, confidence, and self-reliance in order to prevent panic, and to make them able to cope with dangerous and novel situations, such as conducting themselves with dignity in the intrusive white society, or surviving on a drifting ice-floe.

PART III

The forward look and the backward glance

CHAPTER 8

New horizons

CULTURAL CHANGE AND HEALTH PROGRAMMES

Health workers and others who are not social scientists often seem to think that cultural studies in depth of a particular community over-emphasize traditional practices and attitudes, and give an impression of cultural continuity being stronger than and resistant to cultural changes. This assessment of contemporary studies of changing rural communities is often made by the health worker with a programme to put across in what he regards as a stubbornly conservative community. He grasps at any evidence he can find of changing ideas among the people and of a willingness to accept new practices, and is impatient with the social scientist who, when studying such communities and the impact of health programmes on them, tries to keep some sort of balance in assessing the socio-economic effects of change. Only a sense of perspective in such studies will provide guide-lines about why the community accepts some or all of the programme and rejects other parts or the whole of it.

When studying social structure and relationships and cultural patterns the anthropologist is concerned to find out which kinds of new contact and which types of change are more or less superficial, such as changes in dress fashions, and which are penetrating deeply into people's emotional life, stirring up new desires and modifying their patterns of thought and action in the general direction of raising their standards of living.

THE PROBLEM OF ISOLATED RURAL COMMUNITIES

The types of rural community that have been used as illustrations in this book stretch through a very long spectrum – all the way from isolated groups, 'villages beyond the end of the road', to villages on a road leading to nearby urban centres, and in between these two extremes are communities with communications and transport facilities of every degree of ease and difficulty. Rural communities within reach of urban centres are the type most familiar to the majority of health workers, who have seldom the time or the opportunity to penetrate farther afield. For this reason it is important to re-emphasize the existence in many parts of the world of large numbers of people who are still cut off from most modern contacts. It is important, too, for the study of changing attitudes to recall the characteristics of those isolated communities referred to in the Introduction: the necessity for self-reliance; the lessons of survival learned from wresting a living from a hostile environment; the confidence as well as the lethargy inherent in old ways of living; the habitual health and hygiene practices which perpetuate communicable and disabling diseases; the existence of barriers, both physical and ideological, to communication of new ideas and acceptance of new services.

A combination of physical isolation and the necessity for self-reliance created problems for the health educators in the South Pacific island areas. The participants in a training course on health education found themselves posing the following fundamental questions, questions that have been echoed in areas that are not small islands, and that arise essentially from lack of communications with the outside world:

'How can you influence people living in rural areas to get water from safe sources? How can you overcome the resistance of people to modern medicine? How can we educate the public that sanitary hygiene plays a big part in the prevention of leprosy and other contagious and infectious diseases? How can we influence people to change their present unsatisfactory village sites to more healthy ones?' (Brown, 1957, p. 16.)

BREAKING THROUGH THE BARRIERS

A breakthrough of the barriers to communication and mobility is taking place, sometimes slowly and sometimes rapidly, as contacts with the outside world open up. Roads, bicycles, trucks and buses, radio, mobile cinema, and mobile clinic – all these are agents of change once the isolation of an area has been overcome. An example of how one man with a bicycle changed the diet of a village shows that changes, in this case of food habits, can come from within peasant societies as well as from outside (Gerlach, 1963).

The people of the Digo tribe, living on the coastal strip of Kenya, had a traditional aversion to eating fresh fish, though they occasionally

86

ate a very little dried fish instead of their usual relish of wild greens. A young man from a village twelve miles inland went away to work in a coastal town and saved enough money to buy a bicycle which he planned to use to build up a trading business. He had seen Indians and Europeans on the coast eating fresh fish, and his idea was to buy fresh fish at the coast and take it on his bicycle to sell in his village. At the beginning he could get very little response, and he lost a good few shillings on his first trips. But he persevered and gave away some fresh fish free to his relatives, and his wife circulated among the village women, telling them how much easier fresh fish is to prepare than wild greens. He and his wife also used the incentive of prestige, saying that fresh fish is the regular diet of wealthy Europeans and Indians in the towns, while village people are 'like animals and eat grass'.

The women in this village began to yield to the attractions of a continuous supply of fish brought to their doors. They found that they saved time formerly spent hunting for wild greens and preparing them for cooking as relish to the staple cereal dish of maize or cassava. The men grumbled that they had to give their wives more money for housekeeping, and tried to argue that greens were vital for good health and 'power'. The women won out, however, and began to ridicule their husbands if they withheld money to buy fish, until it became a matter of prestige among village families to avoid eating greens more than once a week. The wives also played on the strong slave complex among the Digo, and accused their husbands of treating them as slaves if they had to go out into the bush to collect greens more than once a week.

SIGNIFICANCE OF BREAKTHROUGH FOR RURAL COMMUNITIES

The writer has found in several countries that bicycles in a village have marked a turning-point towards new practices and ideas. The same is true of the radio, whether owned privately by householders or installed in some public spot in a village where people congregate to listen. One report (Loison, 1960) tells of a health education programme on the building and use of latrines in a French African village on the Congo River, where hookworm was said to be very prevalent among the children. The medical officer first made contact with the mothers in the maternal and child health clinic by asking them what their babies suffered from most, and when they replied 'fever', he arranged for a weekly distribution of Nivaquine to all preschool children. Then he went to the school and had a lively quiz with the children, finally asking, 'Is it better to relieve yourself in the bush like the animals, or in a pit which is a latrine?' No one chose the pit, and some added, 'You can fall in.' The teacher realized that his hygiene lessons were having very little effect. With the doctor's help his lessons were then recast and the medical aide came with a microscope to show the eggs and larvae of hookworm.

The next step was a school hygiene committee and a programme of cleaning up the village on Saturdays. The pupil who was top of his class was 'President' of the school committee, and all the school helped to dig a *cabinet d'honneur* in his father's compound. This was the beginning of a steady, even if slow, programme of extending the building and use of latrines. Every week, however, in a radio talk to the area the doctor mentioned this village by name, and named the 'President' of the school committee, the medical aide, and the teacher. The radio publicity stirred up pride in the villagers and elsewhere evoked a desire to emulate them.

First the roads, then the bicycles, then the radio – these may act like a tidal wave that finally breaks and floods an area and its people with a new consciousness of goals to be reached and possible steps to be taken towards them. The making of roads is far more than a symbol of the end of isolation. Access to markets and opportunities of trading provide new incentives for production, and, like access to water supplies in their fields, increased production gives villagers a sense of escape from the narrow limits of their former existence. This sense of an escape from fate is the first stage of breaking the vicious circle of poverty, hunger, and ill health. To people whose cycle of work and subsistence economy formerly depended entirely on monsoon rains with all their irregularities, the provision of extended irrigation and, even more, of electric field pumps brings the wholly new prospect of using their land to produce two and more crops a year. Buying pumps on a hire-purchase system in parts of Bihar, India, caught on so quickly that the demand for pumps soon outran the possibilities of supply. Any surplus cash formerly set aside for investing in jewellery was now set aside for regular payments on the pumps.

Some of these basic problems were discussed with the writer by the director and staff of the Qalyub Research Centre near Cairo, when the importance of understanding the 'climate of opinion' among village people was constantly referred to. The director emphasized again and again that in many rural areas people lived in an environment offering many hazards and few resources. In their present struggle for existence their greatest need was to be able to look forward to a better level of living. An appeal to them to change their food and health habits generally fell on deaf ears, because they were so well aware of their own insecurities and so used to them that they had in the past made all the adjustments that seemed possible. Hence they appeared uncertain and sceptical about new proposals to alter their way of living. Yet suggestions about new uses of their existing resources, and particularly evidence of some small successes, might make them aware of the possibility of escape from the ceaseless effort to achieve a bare existence.

The psychological experience of an escape from a fatalistic acceptance of a perennial shortage of food supplies (and its consequent contraction of the horizon of possibilities) introduces a second profound psychological change for communities newly released from isolation and self-sufficiency. These communities now have before them a range of choices, hitherto outside their grasp. People in the lower economic levels of these communities can base their choices on emulating the standards of living of better-off families, and they may also choose to respond to one or more of the persuasive programmes of health, agricultural, and other improvement services.

CHOICE OF PRIORITIES IN RESPONSE TO HEALTH PROGRAMMES

Examples from Mexico

Two examples from Mexico illustrate the selective process of choice in people's acceptance or rejection of new ideas.

In a small island community in western Mexico a programme to develop cooperatives centred on better chickens and bees, and the increased sales of the produce awakened new interests among the people.[1] The villagers began to talk among themselves about the advice given to them to improve their poultry. The cooperative officer heard them saying that the chickens were good teachers: if chickens are vaccinated, they do not die, so why not have the children vaccinated also? They were impressed by the kind of foodstuffs that they saw were put into the prepared concentrates for chicken feed: fish, dried milk,

---

[1] Personal communication.

meat, maize, etc. They said among themselves, 'If this is good for chickens, perhaps it is good also for humans.' In a rural health and welfare programme in another part of Mexico (Kelly, 1954), classes offered in cooking and nutrition were ignored by the poorer members of the community. These same people expressed to the anthropologist a keen interest in learning to dress-make, to 'do addition', 'tell the time by the clock', and read and write. Literacy classes asked for by the poorer people were a success and proved to be the beginning of an interest in improving diets.

An example from Japan

A demonstration project in public health in Japan (Miyasaka, 1962) also brought out how the villagers use their new-found opportunities of selection and choice, and how their choices do not always coincide with the initial objective of the planners. In one area a Health Council set up to advise the head of the village showed excellent organization on paper, but did not function as planned. In this project there was cooperation up to 75 per cent in vaccination and in an annual faecal examination, but only a limited number took part in adult TB screening. The interest of the people, particularly in the low-income families, was in economic improvement and the education of their children. Most of the villagers were interested in fly and mosquito control, control of acute communicable diseases, and a good water supply; but not in nutrition or maternal and child health, though the physique of the schoolchildren was not good, and their height and weight were below the Japanese average. Housewives consulted among themselves and cooperated actively in a campaign to save money for a new waterworks because they felt that this was urgently necessary for their community. A second later survey of people's interests in this Japanese village showed the following priorities: housing, education, agricultural mechanization, fly and mosquito control. It was noticeable that when women were in control of and managing the domestic economy, the general level of living steadily improved.

The new choices due to the greater accessibility of towns and wayside stores and markets bring the sale of patent medicines near to village people. Increased sales of liniments, cough mixtures, worm tablets, as well as 'cure-all' remedies are reported from many areas. This, as reported from a Central American area,[1] can create an attitude of

[1] Personal communication.

resignation towards illness and a reliance on pills and injections as the only remedies. There is often a corresponding inertia about improving hygiene and cleanliness.

IMPLICATIONS OF THESE PRIORITIES FOR HEALTH WORKERS

When rural people show a desire to improve their level of living in ways chosen by themselves, in many parts of the world their first step is to improve their houses. This is to them a symbol of prestige as well as a chance of living more comfortably. It can also be a new and valuable line of cooperation with health programmes. New housing affords an opportunity for health workers to put across effective programmes for hygiene in the home, and particularly to make provision for individual household latrines. Better houses are a status symbol. So is the acquisition of a transistor or radio set. Public health workers can make effective use of the household or loud-speaker radio to encourage new efforts at household hygiene, and enlist cooperation in their programmes.

EXAMPLES OF VILLAGERS' COOPERATION IN
PUBLIC HEALTH PROGRAMMES

Village sanitation in North India

Experienced health personnel in India, who are battling with problems of sanitation in villages, recognize that building a new and better house is one of the best methods of introducing a household latrine. In so many villages the existing house structure, especially in the poorer and crowded parts of the village, makes the installation of individual house latrines very difficult, and public latrines, except in a very few areas, are not popular. In an orientation centre for rural health medical personnel in North India, the trainees were taught to make maps of villages, showing the types of house in the village and their location. This gave the health workers a realistic approach to the difficulties of village sanitation, and at the same time introduced them to the possibility of utilizing the incentive for better housing, arising from the villagers' hopes of bettter living.

Housing and health education in Ceylon

A study of housing programmes in Ceylon (Karunaratne and Ganewatte, 1964) carried out by the health services drew attention to the

desire of the people to have better houses as economic conditions improved, and to have houses made of more permanent materials, since
this is a symbol of prestige. Many cultural beliefs about house-building
were examined, such as the need for 'auspicious' days on which to
begin the work, and to move into the house; the 'house-warming'
ceremony; the first meal cooked in the house to be given to the priests;
and so on. The study revealed that though many village people today
understand that food, water, and disposal of excreta are causes of
disease, yet they do not realize the connexion between good housing
and good health.

A health education pilot project in Ceylon (Ganewatte, 1962) carried
out in an area where the economic level of the people was low and there
was much indebtedness, brought out clearly the connexion between
improved economic conditions and a new awareness of health problems.
The six stages of this project illustrate not only the relation between
health education and economic advance but also the way in which a
village community took hold of a project initiated from outside and
directed it towards their own desired ends.

Stage I was the presentation to a mass rally of villagers of a survey
made in the village. This was made a gay occasion with music and
dancing, and there was an exhibition of the results of the survey, including demographic data, kinds of houses, showing those that had flies,
mosquitoes, bugs, etc., ventilation, water storage, latrines, manure pits,
and so on.

Stage II was the presentation by the people to the health personnel
of what they considered the chief community needs: a road to the
village, a bus service and a post office; bathing facilities; improvements
to the cemetery; a milk centre and better nutrition for children; a
public health midwife and a government dispensary; recreation
facilities for the young men; de-worming of children; and more latrines.

In Stage III they developed and discussed their needs and classified
them into problems that could be solved by self-help and problems that
would require government assistance. In the first category came a
textile-weaving centre, a bathing well, latrines, vaccination, de-worming, the cemetery, the market-place, the cleaning of the local stream,
and a drive to boil drinking water. Government help was needed for
the dispensary, the midwife, the milk centre, the road and the bus
service, a bridge, and training in poultry-rearing and fruit-growing.

Stage IV was the organization of work camps in which most people gave free labour, rich people gave free food, religious leaders supported and blessed the drive, and communal work was done on holidays and full-moon nights.

Stage V was an assessment of work done after one year. A textile-weaving centre had been set up and twenty-five young girls were learning weaving. Land had been given for the centre by one villager, and another had given land for the bathing well. So many latrines had been constructed that the public health inspector reported that the demand for cement was difficult to cope with. A reading room had been set up, many vaccinations given, and almost all households were boiling their drinking water. Government personnel on their side had arranged for the visiting dispensary, the midwife, the milk centre, and the necessary training.

Stage VI showed three significant developments. The leadership of the village had changed and young men were now members of the working committee. The villagers themselves made annual evaluation surveys. After the project was under way there were no reported cases of typhoid, dysentery, or major communicable diseases.

The most important of all the results of this pilot project is the progressive increase in the cooperation of the villagers in public health programmes. This was achieved, as the description of the project makes clear, by inviting the people to make their own suggestions about improving conditions in the village, even though many of the suggestions (such as the post office and the weaving centre) had apparently little connexion with health. The project presents a clear demonstration of the wholeness of village life, as well as of people's willingness to cooperate in health programmes if their other more strongly felt needs can be met.

Introduction of safe water supplies

After better homes as the first stage in a new level of living, the next step in people's demands is often for a convenient and safe water supply for domestic use, one that ensures freedom from contamination and relieves the housewife from the burden of carrying water long distances. In a village survey carried out by the Health Education Bureau in Lucknow, India (Bharara, 1962), forty-nine out of fifty people knew that contaminated water caused cholera, typhoid, and dysentery, and all the households wanted either properly constructed wells or hand pumps for safe water supplies. The writer has seen piped water brought to villages in Malaya, Mexico, and elsewhere, but though its benefits and convenience are readily acknowledged, not all households are willing to pay for water to be laid on in their house or compound. It takes time for the idea of paying for water to be accepted by householders, accustomed to fetch it from a spring or well or stream or tank. As an intermediate stage, several taps in a village at convenient points lighten the load of housewives, and it is easier to send children to fetch the water from a tap than from a well.

A case report from Yugoslavia (Marković, 1962) dealt with health education in relation to water supplies and sanitation. In a town in Yugoslavia which had had a series of typhoid epidemics, a campaign was launched for voluntary inoculation against typhoid. Among younger people and schoolteachers there was 90 per cent response, but among the rest of the adults the response was nearer 50 per cent, a reflection, it was thought, of the fact that typhoid was no longer a killing disease. On the other hand, the people's committee of the community after prolonged consultations decided to find the necessary money to install some effective waterworks, so that the water would be purified before it reached the houses. The same willingness to find money to install an improved water supply in Tonga has been reported (Spillius, 1962).

AMBIVALENCE OF PEOPLE'S RESPONSE

Evaluation studies in several areas indicate the beginnings of cooperation by village people in health programmes. They also show evidence of resistance to some types of programme, and of a general indifference to the scientific reasons put forward for the programmes. What is clear from the studies already made is that in rural areas, once contact is made and the vicious circle is broken enabling a new future to open up, village people are not slow to decide their own priorities. These priorities concern first an improvement in the economic level of living, and then the provision of long-felt needs such as a water supply and roads.

Where a better level of living is only envisaged but not yet assured the natural fear of taking risks with slender resources is still prevalent:

'Evidence (from China, India and Latin America) indicates that many technological development programs, including medical programs, have failed because the economic margin of the recipients was so slight they would not risk what little security they enjoyed by trying new and untested procedures' (Foster, 1958, p. 22).

A re-survey of a North Indian village after thirty years' work showed that the village people

'are now discovering that something better than they have ever known is within their reach. They want it. But experience with its harsh lessons has made them shrewd in their appraisal of anything unfamiliar that is offered to them. It has taught them not to let go easily of the little they have. And the poorer they are, the more wary they must be. The result is that while they are reaching out for the new opportunities with one hand, they are keeping a firm grip on the old supports with the other' (Wiser, 1963, p. 160).

And in Egypt:

'Through long-established familiarity with their own practices they have achieved a certain sense of security in the so-called "insecurities" as judged from our point of view' (Ammar, 1960, p. 10).

CHAPTER 9

Drugs, injections, and opening doors

DEVELOPMENTS INFLUENCING ATTITUDES TO HEALTH PROGRAMMES

As rural populations emerge from their isolation and begin to see beyond the horizon of a bare struggle for existence, several new developments influencing their attitudes to health programmes can be traced.

The first is the systematic planning and operation of campaigns to control and eventually to eradicate certain endemic diseases. This is one method by which contacts are being made and health programmes are reaching more and more communities in remote areas. The dramatic success of treatment with certain drugs (injections are especially popular) makes a lasting impression when they are used to clear up a long-standing, disabling, disease recognized as such by the people. This success in turn opens doors for other health services. The second development is the effect of better economic standards of living, especially improved water supplies, housing, and sanitation, on helping to clear up certain diseases. The third development is the successful treatment of some diseases at certain stages by chemotherapy, which can be carried out by the people themselves, thus avoiding long residence in hospital and overcrowding of clinics.

Yaws campaigns

The 'opening door' effect of yaws control has been emphasized in several WHO publications A monograph points out that, in those places where yaws is highly prevalent, its social and economic implications are so apparent that the work of health education is already well under way almost spontaneously. A yaws-control campaign is a good method for stimulating general health services because the disease is relatively easy to diagnose and the treatment expectations are good (WHO, 1953, pp. 348, 356).

At the second Asian yaws conference in Bandung, illustrations were given of the effects of better levels of living on the success of yaws-control campaigns. Yaws in Ceylon has reached a near-eradication stage not only through intensive patient treatment with arsenical preparations from 1922 to 1935 but also by the spread of education, health facilities, and the improvement of socio-economic factors such as irrigation works, new roads, and the wide use of soap. In the Philippines the mass campaign against yaws has been made a part of the public health structure of the country and has been integrated into the large network of rural health units since 1954. In Thailand a 'watch' is kept on the most susceptible groups in the community, namely those under fifteen years of age. The school thus becomes the unit of operation, not only for yaws surveillance but also for other preventive measures, such as smallpox vaccination and the treatment of common skin diseases or acute bacterial conjunctivitis.

In East Nigeria also a successful yaws campaign became an opening door to the extension of general health services. Thirty rural health centres were set up in the areas which had been covered by the campaign. The local district councils mobilized communal labour, and contributed building materials and financial aid, which in some cases covered the total cost of the centres. This spontaneous action reflects the attitude of the local people, who saw the effects of the yaws campaign and proceeded, through this self-help measure, to ensure that other health services would be available to them in these rural centres – services which they are now aware that they need.

In the Pacific the same kind of follow-up by the local people took place in the Solomon Islands, where, after the yaws campaign, the villagers demanded visits by health personnel to give them curative services. In Samoa it became a matter of national pride that the country should be completely free of yaws, and as a result of propaganda on these lines the people cooperated well with the follow-up work.

Malaria control

One of the programmes that are reaching farther and farther into remote rural areas is the malaria-eradication and control campaign. The writer was impressed in India with the sense of release from recurrent fever expressed by villagers in many areas as a result of the malaria-control programmes. This new-found freedom leads in many cases to greater willingness to cooperate with other health programmes. In one area successful malaria control is having the effect of rousing the people to make many demands for health services in other fields. The village people are beginning to realize their responsibility in cooperating with control programmes. From another part of India it was reported that the people are keenly interested in the activities of the malaria survey worker, keep an eye on what he does, and complain to the health authorities if he fails to visit the village at regular intervals.

Not all the reactions to malaria campaigns are favourable. In some parts of India, as in other countries, the villagers have been known to lock up their houses and refuse to have them sprayed because spraying greatly increases the bed-bug nuisance. A change made in the chemical spray mixture reduced the bed-bug nuisance and the villagers became more ready to cooperate.

Mention was made earlier of a study of reactions to malaria campaigns in Orissa (Dhillon and Karm, 1961). The tribal people were half-hearted about cooperating with the spraying activities of the malaria-eradication programme for several reasons. One was that they do not regard poor health as one of their major problems. If government wants to send people to help them, then what they want is more irrigation, more roads, better drinking water, rather than the spraying of their houses. Mosquitoes, like bed bugs, are annoying, but not harmful. Malaria, thought to be due to climatic changes during the hot weather and the rains, is regarded as a relatively minor problem because, with time, the fever goes down by itself. Though villagers accept the spraying operations, for fear that they might be prosecuted for resisting, they dislike them because they increase bed bugs, make the rooms smell bad, spoil the coloured plaster of the walls, and make it necessary to move all the furniture.

Some of the same reasons for unwillingness to cooperate with spraying activities are reported from Surinam. The villagers dislike moving their furniture, especially if the team fails to turn up on the appointed day. Cockroaches, which are a greater nuisance than mosquitoes in the interior, increase as a result of spraying. Sometimes chickens, cats, and puppies are killed. People are afraid that their food or the animals' feed will be contaminated, and that wall clocks and radios will be spoiled. There is a general tendency among villagers to wait and see what neighbours are going to do and then to follow suit. Anthropologists working in the area have suggested that before spraying begins it would be better to find out what real health problems the villagers are aware of and perhaps try to solve them first.

In Mexico, eradication is complete except in about 25 per cent of the malarious areas where control is evading spraying. The women cooperate well with the spraying, which they prefer to the mass treatment by pills. The men resist treatment by pills more than the women and are afraid of its effects on their virility. It was found that if the men refuse to take the drugs the whole family follows suit; and if influential men in the village refuse, the whole village follows them. In order to get greater cooperation, efforts were made to enlist voluntary helpers to clear up these last reservoirs of malaria, to distribute pills, and to take blood slides. Furthermore, the radio was called into play for broadcasts twice a month, for transistors are found in many of the poorest homes where there is nothing else of value.[1]

In the Sudan an evaluation study was made after a health education programme in malaria control had been carried out in two villages in the Gezira, where the population of both villages had been semi-nomadic before they were resettled (Babiker and Beshir el Sheikh, 1962). The survey was a pilot study to find out how best to plan health education in order to get the fullest cooperation from the villagers. The people were asked about the cause and symptoms of malaria and the habits of mosquitoes. After the health education programme, still 31 per cent and 37 per cent did not know respectively the cause and the symptoms of malaria, but knowledge about mosquitoes' habits increased so that 70 per cent knew their breeding places, 89 per cent the breeding season, and 87 per cent the results of spraying and killing mosquitoes. At first in both villages there was a general unwillingness to allow blood slides to be taken from children under one year. After the programme there was 100 per cent attendance for slide-taking, since attendance was associated with the issue of multivitamin tablets for the children.

Treatment of trachoma

The relation between general standards of living and hygiene and disease is illustrated by the case of trachoma, 'the single greatest cause of serious and progressive loss of sight'. The following quotation indicates the nature of this relationship:

'Trachoma becomes endemic only where there exist widespread environmental factors favoring transmission of infection. . . . History has repeatedly shown that trachoma disappears from a community with improvements in standards of living and hygiene, and conversely, that if these standards are too low, treatment of cases (on

[1] Personal communication.

any scale that is practicable) may have little effect in reducing the incidence of the disease. . . . From existing evidence, which is largely circumstantial, it would seem that levels and changes, both in prevalence and in severity, may be dependent more upon environmental factors than on differences in host susceptibility or in viral strains. . . . Under the worst conditions of poverty, overcrowding and squalor it has not been possible with present day treatment methods to make any substantial reduction in the incidence of trachoma. Hundreds of thousands of cases have been cured and a high proportion saved from the disastrous end results of the disease, but new cases continue to appear in almost equal numbers' (Lyons, 1960).

An anthropological study was made in the Qalyub area in Egypt in February 1960 to find out the extent to which communicable eye diseases are regarded by the community as important health problems, the attitude of the people towards these infections, and their usual behaviour regarding them (Attiah, El Kholy, and Omran, 1962). The health authorities considered the study valuable for two reasons: because human behaviour is an important causal factor in the occurrence of these diseases; and because the research would provide essential background knowledge for planning a health-education campaign. The study followed an earlier mass-treatment campaign for trachoma, and was intended to check upon the effects of treatment in a selected community. One clear result emerged, namely that a change was taking place in people's ideas about the nature of and treatment for trachoma. References to 'folkloric treatment' were made mainly by the older age group. The causes of the disease were given by the schoolchildren as: dirt, dust, going barefoot, flies; and by the older people as: fate, dirt, going barefoot, eating salty food. The policy in planning and carrying out campaigns against trachoma is to use volunteer helpers in order to get the people to feel that they are sharing in the project.

In the Sudan the public health aspect of trachoma was recognized by the health authorities and a pilot survey was carried out in an area where there was a prevalence of over 24 per cent of severe cases, rising to 71 per cent in one village; and where one in four of the population had a fair degree of disability due to permanent eye irritation. Although the survey team chose economically poor quarters of towns for the study, it was found that there was more trachoma and more severe trachoma in villages than in nearby towns, presumably because in the latter there is easier access to medical care and to water supplies. The incidence of active trachoma was found to be higher among children than among adults, and among women than among men, since men have few direct contacts with infected children. The application of antibiotics was carried out by 'local leaders', sheikhs, merchants, farmers, and some senior women, all of whom had some training before and during the treatment period, especially in methods of approaching and educating the local population and the schoolchildren.

Treatment of tuberculosis

The quick response of certain diseases to modern treatment by drugs and injections may win the people's support for health programmes whether they grasp the nature of the disease and its scientific cause or not. Tuberculosis among the Navaho yielded dramatically to chemotherapy. On the other hand, a more reluctant attitude to treatment and less willingness to cooperate were found among a rural population in Uganda.[1] There the people believe firmly that tuberculosis comes through 'poisoned' food or drink that has been made harmful by people of ill will. They also refuse to accept the fact that a tuberculous mother can infect her own child, because no mother would ever wish her child ill. Nevertheless, they recognize that some children improve with medical treatment, and hence they usually go to the hospital for advice.

In Egypt, around the Qualyub demonstration centre, a tuberculosis survey by mass radiography was carried out covering the entire population over five years of age. The fullest possible cooperation of the people was desired by the promoters of the project, and it was successful in getting 95 per cent of the population to come for examination. The project was first discussed with the leaders in each village, who were asked to assign a place where the x-ray apparatus could be set up, and their cooperation was uniformly good. When treatment followed examination the policy was to give dried skim milk and flour to all individuals each time they came for treatment, partly in order to encourage them to come regularly, and partly because the improvement that follows treatment makes people very hungry. Also, some cases had to take time off to rest as part of the treatment and therefore could not work for their food and livelihood.[2]

Some advance in the acceptance of modern medical treatment

[1] Personal communication.   [2] Personal communication.

and preventive measures is due to the recognition by the people themselves of the symptoms of certain diseases. If a patient can describe
his symptoms specifically and accurately the physician is much assisted
in his diagnosis and treatment. A study was carried out in South India,
by a physician who was also a sociologist working with a non-medical
sociologist, to investigate the awareness of symptoms among cases of
pulmonary tuberculosis (Banerji and Anderson, 1962). The study was
also related to the public health aspect of tuberculosis treatment in a
future programme aimed eventually at control. In a pre-pilot study
phase, social investigators were first trained in the techniques of inter-
viewing. They then interviewed large numbers of villagers in Mysore
State on what they thought their health problems were; how many
villagers were going to towns to work and returning to the villages;
and what were thought to be symptoms of tuberculosis. The inter-
viewers found that the villagers on the whole liked to talk about their
health, and were glad to know that someone was taking an interest in
their wellbeing.

When the pilot study was launched in thirty-nine random selected
villages and towns, 2,000 persons, known TB cases and controls, were
interviewed to determine how many had symptoms suggestive of TB.
All types of symptoms given by the people were recorded, including
headache and sore eyes, but only persons reporting cough or fever
for one month and more, pain in the chest, or blood in the sputum were
considered symptomatic and were examined.

The planners of the study worked on the assumption that among the
peasants and townspeople there are three levels of consciousness or
awareness of symptoms. The first is a rather vague consciousness of the
presence of one or more symptoms; the second they called a 'worry
awareness', because awareness of one or more symptoms is a source of
worry and anxiety to the sufferer; the third is an acute kind of awareness
that makes the sufferer take action and seek treatment. On the whole,
men reported symptoms more often than women, especially quite
young and very old women. Awareness at the second level was found in
70 per cent of the sputum positive cases and in 80 per cent of the radio-
logically active cases.

The conclusion from the study is that it would be epidemiologically
and economically justified, in present circumstances in India, to base
the tuberculosis control programme on cases seeking treatment motivated by worry over symptoms. When the services satisfying the needs

of the already worried tuberculosis cases are well developed, then mass case-finding can be embarked on as an additional measure. The eventual aim is to integrate the tuberculosis programme with the existing health services; and this is associated with the general problem of the restitution of disabled persons to a normal working life.

REHABILITATION AFTER ILLNESS

In a rural economy which is neither diversified nor advanced, the reabsorption of individuals after treatment into their own community poses a number of socio-economic problems. Some of these were discussed at the first WHO Expert Committee on Medical Rehabilitation (WHO, 1958), which defined the aims of medical rehabilitation as the achievement of not only a physical but a social cure, restoring the individual to self-reliance in daily life, treating him as 'a whole and not as an assortment of organs and extremities'. It was recognized that much health education is needed, especially in countries where there is a prejudice against handicapped persons, or where the population has little understanding of the potentialities after successful treatment of an individual whom they always associate with dependency and inability to work. The committee found a close relation between preventive health measures, as in communicable eye diseases, and the subsequent treatment and rehabilitation of persons who had lost their sight through neglect of early symptoms.

The reabsorption into their communities of former sufferers from diseases which are greatly feared, such as leprosy and tuberculosis, constitutes a problem in health education of a particularly difficult type, for the reasons just given. In no field is this seen more clearly than in the field of mental health.

Recent research has brought out the fear of the general community in respect of those suffering from acute mental illness, which can present a terrible and disrupting element in normal social life. The acceptance or rejection of mentally ill persons depends, however, partly on the patient and his symptoms, but also on the beliefs of the society about the symptoms of mental abnormality and on its criteria for a 'normal personality'. Tolerance, as opposed to fear, of mentally ill persons depends upon a culturally determined view of normal behaviour, and still more on the concepts of the origin and nature of abnormal behaviour. In some cultures mentally ill persons are considered dangerous and even evildoers, and there is a widespread tendency to get rid of such people out of the community, and put them under restraint or under treatment. But where mental patients are withdrawn and not violent, the community may tolerate them and even show protectiveness towards them. In the Lebanon, where elderly people in a house are considered to bring a blessing to the household, the tendency is that, when housing conditions permit, both normal and abnormal old people are taken care of at home.

In a discussion of rehabilitation related to psychiatric treatment, and in particular of the Aro (Nigeria) hospital scheme for boarding out mental health patients in neighbouring villages, the authors (Leighton and Lambo, 1963) speak of the way in which traditional religious leaders play a conspicuous part in the psychotherapeutic management of some patients. They state that patients treated in a community setting often fail to develop certain symptoms which are apparently induced by hospital situations. The success of such boarding-out treatment has been found to depend on the nature of the village environment and the village social structure. The experience of placing patients, accompanied by a relative or two, in a nearby village to attend for outpatient treatment at the hospital has been built up on a selected kind of village community. The village should have a viable, relatively harmonious social organization, active and responsible leadership, and not too rapid socio-economic change. The village leaders met monthly with the senior hospital staff, and they received some financial assistance in developing water supplies, pit latrine construction, and mosquito eradication. The village setting was used as a therapeutic milieu where the patients could be with one or more relatives, be accepted in the village community, and earn small sums and a new self-respect by doing what work was possible, such as selling vegetables, washing clothes, weaving, etc.

SOCIAL STRUCTURE IN RELATION TO HEALTH PROGRAMMES

Forms of treatment that enlist the cooperation of many people in the community, such as the trachoma village treatments and the boarding-out of some kinds of mental patients, can constitute an opening door for changing attitudes towards preventive health services and for health education. Recent research has shown, however, that much depends on the nature and stability of the social structure in rural communities.

Health workers and social scientists have drawn attention to the relevance of the traditional social structure of a community. This may be well integrated, with acknowledged leaders in positions of responsibility; or it may be faction-ridden, with deep-seated sectional interests militating against combined action. Illustrations of how social structure could assist health programmes occurred in the study of water supplies in Tonga (Spillius, 1962), and in the organization of trachoma campaigns in the Sudan. The pilot study in Ramanagram in Mysore (see p. 50 above) showed how the statutory position of the village headman was effective in reporting communicable diseases to the health inspector. It showed also how non-statutory bodies such as 'Health Leagues' functioned. The Health Leagues were encouraged by health centres to involve the community in their own health problems such as water supplies, cattle sheds, village cleanness, etc. In the study in Orissa (Dhillon and Karm, 1961) the social scientist emphasized that the well-knit village structure of the tribal groups was a promising factor in getting the people's cooperation, since there were few factional rivalries. The traditional village head was the liaison between the people and the government, and he was as a rule receptive to new ideas and proud of his knowledge of the outside world.

CHAPTER 10

Channels of new ideas about health and sickness

The health planner and administrator, the physician, the public health nurse, and the health educator, all alike are concerned to ascertain and assess the effects of changing ideas on people's response to health programmes. In these situations the social scientist finds himself driven to analyse the wider processes of culture change which are taking place in a given area. He tries first to get a general conspectus of directed socioeconomic change which has resulted in certain new practices and ways of living being adopted by a community. He then tries to see health services in terms of new treatments, on the one hand, and health education, on the other. At this point he can trace certain stages in a sequence of cause and effect arising from the initiation of particular health programmes.

STAGES IN ACCEPTANCE OF HEALTH PROGRAMMES

Stage I involves a demonstration of successful modern treatment for a particular disease such as tuberculosis or yaws; a general acceptance by the community of the facilities for such treatment; and a growing conviction on the part of the majority of the community that the treatment is efficacious because sick people have been seen to be cured.

Stage II has two facets. Individuals in a community begin to cooperate with the facilities set up for the treatment and control of localized or endemic diseases and to offer their support for installing and supervising these facilities, as in the case of some of the malaria, yaws, and trachoma programmes. At the same time, influenced by those known successes achieved in Stage I and by the cumulative process of socioeconomic change, they demand from the government more facilities for general curative services, as illustrated in several reports. In the Sudan more demands were being made than could be met from financial resources for dispensaries, health centres, and hospitals. The demands came from populations that not so long ago had burned dispensaries and refused to allow wives to go to antenatal clinics. The change of attitude was attributed partly to the success of medical care in homes and clinics, but also to the fact that people read more, listen to the radio, and travel more. In Mysore the pilot study on local health services showed that people were seeking hospitalization and western medicine more and more. This development was partly the result of local improvements in transport, electrification, education, and employment.

As had been found elsewhere, the pragmatic factor was important in changing Navaho attitudes to medical treatment:

'The medicine men gave up treating TB once they saw that the white man had a more effective cure. In fact, it was not until chemotherapy greatly reduced the period of bed rest, and the Navaho saw their relatives return home completely cured, that they became convinced that the white doctors had a superior cure to their own.

'It should be noted that it was not the scientific explanations of the drug's effect on the tubercle bacillus which turned the tide; it was the demonstrated worth of these drugs, the results of this method of treatment, which convinced the Navaho. . . .

'In other aspects of modern medicine we find acceptance today where there was rejection 20 years ago. Surgery for appendicitis, gall-bladder disease and orthopaedic correction for congenital hip as as well as thoracic surgery for advanced cases of pulmonary TB have all gained acceptance. Today the hospital wards are crowded, whereas a generation ago they were regarded as death traps, haunted by the spirits of the dead' (Adair, 1963).

Stage III, anticipated and hoped for by health planners and health workers, is still in the future, and not only in developing countries. It includes a general acceptance of scientific medical care in all cases of illness, mental as well as physical; and a grasp of some at least of the principles underlying the practice of preventive medicine shown in the willingness of individuals and communities to cooperate with physicians and public health authorities.

Given the significant forms of response from people in Stages I and II, the task for the future is to discover through what channels new ideas about health are reaching rural populations. Evidence from different parts of the world suggests three likely channels. One has already emerged in discussing Stages I and II – namely, the dramatic success of some modern treatments. The second is the rising tide of expectations among rural people about a better standard of living; and the third is the infiltrating though slow influence of modern education of all kinds.

THE RISING TIDE OF EXPECTATIONS

Why should a rising tide of expectations among rural people be a channel through which people become susceptible to new ideas? Perhaps for the first time they have a little surplus of food and can trade with it to make money to buy other necessities. Women may have a little leisure because there is a water supply right in the village. There is a road to the village, and bicycles and buses bring townspeople to them, and villagers can go more easily to the market-place. Women especially can use their new-found money, time, and transport facilities to satisfy new needs. The satisfaction of these needs is frequently influenced by motives of prestige – that desire to emulate someone else's level of living which is often an 'activating element' in people's choice of action. In urban areas it is well known that prestige factors influence women's choice of clothes, house decoration, and food purchases. In the past, societies following a more or less traditional pattern regarded status and prestige as something fixed in the social structure, and persons of status were members of a certain family or clan or caste or ethnic group. Prestige also pertained to authority acquired through age, or to the status of a grandmother or a senior wife. Traditional societies now recognize additional marks of higher status, conferring prestige and commanding respect, such as a person's wealth, or educational level, or public position held. Among some West African societies women, as well as men, achieved a new status with a higher prestige-rating by 'buying themselves into title societies' – an expensive and protracted undertaking. In the Ibo study already referred to (Ottenberg, 1959), the Ibo women were found to be putting their money, formerly spent on 'buying titles', into better homes and improved education for their children. New prestige symbols indicate socio-economic changes, and hence the possessors of the symbols may acquire a new status. The writer knew many African villages where a man who had made money working outside the country used it, on his return, to build a stone or brick house and to give his wife good clothes. The prestige symbols of house and clothes gave the man's wife a new status, which in many cases was not hers by right of birth or age.

An anthropologist working in Pakistan made the following points about the prestige aspects of food and food habits, related to the fact that choice made on grounds of prestige did not always improve the diet. She discussed the differences in diet between rural and city people and the special foods associated with status and prestige. In East Pakistan, for example: 'a gentleman does not eat red rice'; or 'rich people do not eat *dal* (pulse) greens.'

'One informant reports that, in her youth, all members of her family ate daily, the first thing in the morning, a handful of gram sprouts, accompanied by a piece of fresh turmeric. . . . Soaked gram is said to be popular among gymnasts, and it is traditional among the religious sages of East Pakistan. Furthermore, it is said that during religious fasting the body becomes dry and "heated", hence the "cooling" effect of soaked gram is advisable when the fast is broken. . . . Although in folk classification gram sprouts are "cooling", there seems to be no prejudice against them for that reason, and it is said specifically that men, women and children eat the sprouted gram, although as a rule men avoid heavy consumption of "cooling" foods in the belief that sexual potency may be reduced. . . . Several other people from East Pakistan deny all knowledge of soaked gram, and it is pretty evident that the dish is associated with villagers and with families of low economic status' (Kelly, 1960).

Elsewhere the prestige attached to the installing of latrines in villages and houses has been noted:

'In the campaign to achieve more latrines, by voluntary labor, and properly sited for the various sections of a village, an intimate knowledge of village leaders, kinship groupings and rival factions proved as essential to health and community development workers as skill in expounding the germ theory of infection in a way acceptable to their hearers. Nor could they afford to ignore the prestige motive. It was gratifying when one village wrote in large letters across its new latrine: "This is the result of True Learning: Enter and See." But the strong inclination of many villages to site their sanitation beside the main road suggested something other than purely intellectual conviction' (Spens, 1960).

In a who sanitation project in Afghanistan the promoters worked out a type of latrine suitable to local conditions: the farmers could have access to the contents, and the sanitarians could have access to the homes and courtyards to give continuous advice about its sanitary use. The latrines designed became a symbol of better living and were readily accepted, with the result that promiscuous defecation and fly-breeding dropped considerably. At the same time the provision of public baths for men in the mosques, and of washing places with showers for the women, roused great enthusiasm – again as a symbol of improvement – and the villagers were prepared to cooperate with labour and materials.

In a survey after five years of a village sanitation programme in Alaska (Lantis, 1962) it was found that one of the problems in dealing with parasitic infection in the villages derived from the fact that large numbers of sled dogs carried parasites. An attempt to control the number of dogs in order to reduce infection came up against a difficulty in that the number of dogs owned was a status symbol in the villages. On another level, the sanitary aides appointed to carry out the programmes had no prestige standing in the villages and therefore no influence, unless they had recognized family connexions or some acknowledged religious affiliation.

THE EFFECT OF EDUCATION

The new expectations of rural people and the possibility of meeting newly discovered needs are everywhere related not only to economic changes but also to modern education of various kinds – schools, adult education, literacy campaigns, community development. Research is much needed on the ways in which these various forms of education are really affecting people's ideas about health, and influencing them to co-operate with health education and preventive health measures. Most of the evidence seems to show that school education is slow to affect people's beliefs about their bodies and their health.

A study in a North Indian village (Khare, 1963) related the persistence of belief in folk medicine to the ways in which villagers listened to the ideas of people they regarded as 'experts'. It was evident that the channels of communication between the villagers and the public health authorities were not so readily made use of.

'Public health workers and also clinical doctors are once again making efforts to realise the significance of the social character of the village medical system. It may be pointed out that the system of folk-medicine assures the people that (*a*) the system is their own and (*b*) that it provides the people with the "best" and "complete" and "secure" ways of coping with their physical and mental ailments. Modern medicine is looked upon by the people as something foreign to their culture.'

But local and visiting 'experts' had a profound influence on the people's ideas:

'Channels of communication also influence the nature of ideas about illness. Certain houses in the village, irrespective of caste rank, can be marked out as centers for dispersal of various kinds of news, anecdotes and past experience. In addition, there are regular visits of the mendicant singers, Sadhus of Ayodhya, priest friends of the village medicine man and a Muslim exorcist who are sources of information about disease. The new ideas about disease which these agents introduce are greatly appreciated and easily added to the body of previous knowledge. Womenfolk are highly susceptible to these suggestions, to which they attentively listen from behind the doors. If men express contrary ideas about the treatment or nature of a disease, their womenfolk quickly remind the men of the opinion given by local experts on the matter.'

On the other hand, it is evident from the study that there are people in the village whose higher socio-economic position and education make them more aware of and sympathetic to modern medical knowledge. Yet even they are not fully committed to a modern view, for the primary school teacher was said to talk about the efficacy of scientific medicine and public health, though he never disowned either publicly or privately the control of diseases by the established supernatural agencies.

THE TENACITY OF TRADITIONAL CONCEPTS

The conservative forces had their way when a vaccinator came to the village to prevent a cholera epidemic, and not more than ten people agreed to be inoculated. The villagers were quick to assert that epidemics are not checked by inoculation because 'an epidemic is air'. This kind of illness could not be bound and controlled except through the great supernatural powers.

The reference to the role of the primary school teacher in the North Indian village suggests that, though school education may be considered by many health workers as an effective channel of communication, in fact the new ideas about health and hygiene taught by the teacher, but often not applied by him, have to compete with the traditional ideas held by the majority of the village people. Some caution therefore is needed when estimating the results of modern schooling on people's ideas and practices about health. Contemporary health problems in advanced countries have shown clearly that universal education is no sure road to a scientific acceptance of preventive health practices. Studies of health education activities in schools in several parts of the world show divergent tendencies. On the one hand, school health teaching and health practices in hygienic surroundings can make some impact on the life of the community. Against this has to be set the fact that there are areas where hygiene and health teaching has been going on for a long time with apparently little or no effect on people's ideas and practices in the surrounding communities.

Figure 4 (cf. Read, 1959) suggests that rural schoolchildren have two

Figure 4   COMPETING INFLUENCES ON SCHOOLCHILDREN

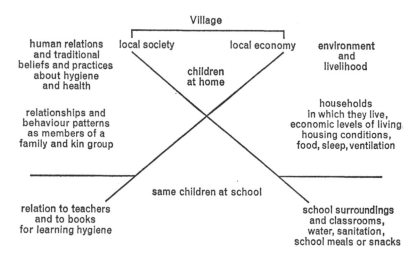

competing sets of influences operating on them, and in a tradition-oriented community the balance may be weighted against what the children learn in school. On the other hand, where community development, literacy campaigns, adult education, the radio in the village, or previous schooling have given parents in a village a new outlook on the possibilities of change of all kinds, this new outlook may well include a desire for the benefits of modern curative medicine, and a dawning consciousness about the importance of preventive action such as immunization, better diet, and environmental sanitation.

In many countries, and by no means only in those called 'developing', ambivalence in attitudes to scientific medicine is well established. People welcome certain health services, are indifferent or hostile to others, and maintain and use their own traditional forms of diagnosis and treatment – all at the same time. An awareness of how these attitudes have arisen and how they work out in practice is of importance to the health worker who is responsible for putting across health programmes.

Evidence is widespread that the acceptance of new practices in medical treatment does not as a rule involve a change of ideas about the causes of illness. For this reason, among others, those who decide to accept new treatments do not thereby abandon all traditional forms of treatment. They may be compelled by the government to undergo vaccination for smallpox, but they may retain at the same time what *they* consider protective measures against the disease. As a result of a study mentioned earlier of public attitudes to smallpox eradication in North India (Bharara, 1962), the Health Education Bureau in their posters and talks emphasized both old and new approaches – i.e. worship the Goddess *and* be vaccinated. The grounds given for this dual approach were that:

'One can scarcely expect village people to change their whole cosmology simply to accord with the outlook of a modern doctor or public health worker. . . . We shall have to accept the inevitable fact that our techniques of cure and prevention will be accepted irrationally.'

In an account of folk medicine in rural Egypt,[1] an Egyptian physician describes the place of modern medicine in rural life. He shows how the spread of health services beyond the towns has made villagers familiar with the scientific names of such diseases as bilharzia, typhoid, and malaria. Visits to clinics are becoming more popular, and when there, rural people ask to be given eye drops, or calcium, or iron, or vitamins. The visit of a doctor to a patient in a village home brings great prestige to a family. But, it is pointed out, though these are new practices for the villagers, the old concepts have not changed. Whatever

[1] Personal communication.

113

new ideas about the efficacy of certain drugs the people acquire are merely added to the old body of knowledge.

An ambivalent attitude towards modern medical services might be regarded as creating additional conflict and stress for the people concerned. This view, however, was rejected by the anthropologist in the case study of the Tiv already quoted. He spoke of his

'participant observation of healing ceremonies, and of his observation and interviews with Tiv attending dispensaries or otherwise attending European doctors. A great deal of enquiry was addressed to the question as to why some Tiv went to European doctors and others did not, and in some circumstances rather than others. To a naive observer it might appear that here there was a conflict choice for Tiv – *akombo* ceremonies on the one hand or European medicine on the other. Responses to questioning failed to elicit any conflict at all. It seemed quite logical for Tiv men and women to go from one to the other or to both at once. This was not a double insurance; it revealed a tendency in Tiv outlook which is fundamental to their understanding of sickness, namely that they conceived of both a volitional and an instrumental causation of illness. Unless the former as well as the latter is satisfied, there is a sense of incompleteness. . . . This attitude, of course, can work both ways, as it can facilitate the working of the new medicine as well as sustain the old. Nevertheless it indicates the process of abstracting a new concept from the matrix of the old. European medicine was certainly effective, Tiv would say . . . but had no real concern with the forces engendering illness. The forces of *akombo* had to be settled. By ascribing a volitional causation, Tiv are able to provide a complicated but satisfying machinery for conflict between kin. Handling illness in an entirely impersonal manner, abstracted from kin and quarrels, there is left a lacuna which for Tiv is unsatisfactory' (Price-Williams, 1962).

THE RELATION BETWEEN PRACTITIONERS AND PATIENTS

Any analysis of how traditional health systems can contribute to modern programmes brings out the fundamental importance of the relation between individual professional health workers and their patients, and the contrast between this relationship and the relationship of traditional practitioners with their clients. This may lie at the roots of much ambivalence.

In a report on a health project in Alaska (Dept of Health and Welfare, 1962) one result of successful health education about the common cold was to establish a sense of dependency on professional health personnel. In this project a very effective learning process took place once the people had grasped the connexion between the common cold and sore throat and incipient or acute ear conditions. The successful treatment given by the health team was, in the eyes of the people, something entirely from outside that bore no relation to their former health practices. The result was that they used the radio to call the doctor for every kind of ailment, doing nothing for themselves. The health team then had to train one or more health aides in each village to take care of the early stages of ear, nose, and throat infections. These people valued good health because their livelihood depended on it, but they had never before recognized that a cold was an illness, or that acute ear infections could develop from neglected colds. The tendency to depend on their kin group in what they considered as illness was transferred to a strong sense of dependency on government medical aid, with the results just described.

In East Nigeria ambivalence showed itself in the way the rural people compared the services of physicians and their own practitioners. An anthropologist among the Anang found that

'it took almost a decade to get the Anang to use the medical resources but today the hospitals are crowded and personnel overworked. Many people regard doctors and dispensers as workers of magic whose skills and medicines gain their efficacy through power dispensed by God and manipulated by the magic spirit, and persons who are ill or have been injured often seek relief from both workers of magic and from doctors. The fact that medicines and hospital treatment cost considerably less than services obtained from Anang practitioners has resulted in a rapidly growing number of people depening almost entirely upon government and mission facilities. It has also forced workers of magic to lower their prices and provide new services, so that only those of high repute or with special skills can charge large enough fees to make their speciality pay; others less famous and those continuing traditional practices are forced to abandon the profession. . . . Recognizing the growing fear of malevolent supernatural forces and spurred by competition from European-trained specialists, workers of magic are resorting to the sale of charms and medicines and abandoning their other pursuits. Indigenous charms are seldom prescribed, for new types are obtained from mail order houses in Europe and America dealing in magical and occult devices; these are thought to be effective, since manufactured and used by people living in Christian countries' (Messenger, 1959, p. 294).

Another aspect of the comparison of the services of physicians and traditional practitioners concerns the attitude of professional and auxiliary health personnel and the atmosphere of modern clinics:

'The instructions in the Quran to "take counsel with them in the affair" for "hadst thou been rough and rude of heart they had dispersed from around" still hold good (El Bedri, 1959). No matter how strong the mother's anxiety, or her desire to see her child's health improve, she cannot but be daunted by an uncongenial atmosphere in the clinic or hospital where she seeks advice. Too much haste, failure to examine the child properly according to the mother's standards, lack of clear and adequate explanations of what she is to do, failure to prescribe medicine for a sick child, and ridicule of the mother's homely remedies are all resented, and militate against the possibility of educating the mother whose child is perhaps on the verge of grave malnutrition' (Burgess, 1960).

In a public health centre in Latin America friction grew between the patients, who came from a depressed slum area, and the middle-class doctors and nurses, because the patients did not understand the organizational working of the clinic (Erasmus, 1961). The doctor ordered the mothers to bring their babies for a regular check-up on what were known as 'well baby days', and threatened to refuse treatment for ill babies unless this regulation was observed. The mothers found these frequent visits very inconvenient and time-consuming, and ceased to come to 'well baby days'. The day came when, carrying out his threat, the doctor refused treatment to sick babies, and bitter feelings were aroused among the women. They contrasted this attitude of the physicians with that of their favourite *curandero*: 'He treats us like people. He is better than a hundred health centres.' They could rely on him to listen to them as they described their symptoms, to prescribe a herbal remedy, and charge no fee.

Egyptian physicians, after reviewing some of the major factors in the difficulty of treating bilharziasis in Egypt, concluded:

'All these factors have resulted in . . . attitudes and patterns of behavior in rural populations which are essentially antagonistic to modern medical practices. On the other hand, native medicine men, lay midwives, barber surgeons and even quacks have been more successful with rural populations. The secret is that such unqualified practitioners had learned by experience the proper approaches to their people. Their sincerity, patience, perseverance, reassuring smiles, soothing words, pleasant attitudes, genuine understanding of the simple psychology of villagers, as well as their human consideration of the weaknesses of people, their prompt response and appearance in time of need, their modesty, all had contributed to their acceptance in the community as celebrated practitioners. They actually enjoy much more confidence and respect than qualified practitioners and this confidence is not shaken by any blunders they made.'[1]

From another source in Egypt (Gadallah, 1962) there is evidence of the benefits derived from a friendly approach from the scientifically trained medical personnel to their patients. Examples are given of how an assistant nurse in a village can approach patients and respond to their offers of hospitality. Physicians, it is suggested, can make use of quotations from the Koran before taking any action, and of proverbs when persuading people to adopt new practices.

There is still much to investigate in the nature of the synthesis or conflict between traditional and modern systems of healing. In advanced as well as in developing countries there is a great gulf between the modern professional health personnel, with their specialized approach to health in the community, and the people themselves, who in the first instance so often rely on uninformed mutual help. It is probably a mistake to expect a scientific outlook from the majority of people in any country, since the distinction in all countries is between the specialists in health and the rest of the people.

[1] Personal communication.

CHAPTER 11

Implications for orientation and training

SOME POSITIVE AND NEGATIVE ELEMENTS IN PEOPLE'S RESPONSE TO HEALTH PROGRAMMES

This book has had two main objectives. The first has been to indicate some ways of discerning the relationship between health programmes and health services and the reactions of the people to these activities. Out of the material presented in the preceding chapters, certain negative elements emerge in the people's response, and some positive ones. The outstanding negative element, one that affects both the planning and the operation of programmes, is that, in many rural areas, health is not a prime concern of the people. This does not mean that they are not concerned about illness. The elaborate protective measures that they have devised for themselves make this very clear. But there is evidence that they have other more dominant concerns, e.g. the possible provision of services such as schools, roads, water supplies. Health personnel should be aware of these interests, because they can make use of them to further health programmes. The second negative element is that rural people in tropical areas have no overall or complete confidence in scientific medicine and its ability to diagnose and treat every kind of complaint. The third negative element, shared by almost all people everywhere, is that they have no concept of health as 'a positive state of wellbeing', in the WHO definition. People who are always underfed, or anaemic, do not know what it is like to feel full of healthy energy and are often not even aware of good health as a possible goal. This profoundly affects attempts to introduce preventive health measures.

Among the positive elements in people's response is their recognition of the efficacy of certain cures achieved by scientifically trained medical and health personnel. This, as we have seen, has led to a rising demand for more curative services in most parts of the world. In a slightly different category, but connected with the first, is the welcome given, especially by the women, to rural health centres established where there was formerly no medical help available. These centres are related

118

to the advent of other services, such as roads, radio, and schools, which break down rural isolation and are evidence to rural people of a new interest taken by governments in their welfare. A third positive element, which has been referred to as opening doors, is the response made to certain, though not to all, control, eradication, and immunization campaigns. This is a particularly notable form of response in view of the prevailing lack of interest in many other preventive health services.

BARRIERS TO COMMUNICATION: IMPLICATIONS FOR TRAINING FOR RURAL HEALTH WORK

The second objective of the book has been to call attention to the barriers to communication between scientifically trained health workers and the public, and to suggest that the social and behavioural sciences might make an important contribution in breaking through these barriers:

'The ethnocentrism of developed societies has led their members to regard those who fail to act in accord with their own practices as being "ignorant" and "superstitious". This has led even specialists to try to contrast the "knowledge" that is to be derived from scientific work, with a thing they call "ignorance" which characterizes most of the world's peoples. This knowledge–ignorance dichotomy is misleading. The significant difference in this matter is not to be found between societies, but between the specialists and the non-specialists. In all societies, most people are non-specialists when it comes to matters of health and nutrition. Although the practices of some societies are clearly more efficacious, as measured in terms of mortality, morbidity and life expectancy, that which the people in those societies "know" about how their own practices work, and how they may react to new practices is quite another matter. So it is that "folk knowledge", and in the present instance specifically folk medicine, has mistakenly been thought to be peculiar to some "ignorant" segments of the world's population when in fact it is a kind of knowledge which characterizes in one way or another almost everyone in the species' (Adams, 1963).

In the training of medical students it is not only the image of the physician as seen by the public that physicians must understand, since everywhere that image dominates the relation of patient to doctor. They have also to be aware of, and increasingly sensitive to, their own professional concept of their role in public health work and of their 'medical culture' which they have acquired through their medical-school training. Problems such as these were discussed at length in a seminar held in Bogotá in February 1964 under the auspices of the Association of Faculties of Medicine of Colombia. The theme of the discussions was 'The social sciences, medical education, and the problems of health of the Colombian community'. Physicians presented problems arising from the social and economic background that were encountered by medical students when they were confronted, especially outside the hospital wards, with the subcultures of remote rural communities or of the economically depressed classes living in the slums of the large cities. Social scientists presented some aspects of environmental and economic hazards to health, the folk-medicine systems of different communities, and the attitude of the public towards traditional practitioners.

The Colombian seminar emphasized two main aspects of the problem of people's response to health programmes. One was concerned with the role of health workers and the problems of communication. Since everyone in rural health services has to assume the role of health educator, whatever his definitive training may have been, it becomes increasingly important that all health workers should acquire some kind of training for this role. Some familiarity with social science concepts and techniques is essential to enable them to recognize the extent and concepts of folk medicine as a first step to overcoming the barriers of communication.

The second emphasis was on the need for medical officers and public health administrators to give a lead in this training. There has been some evidence throughout this book that here and there professional medical personnel are becoming interested in the possibilities of a new approach to rural people and to their traditional folk-medicine practices. The preparation of the physician in all countries was discussed in the World Health Assembly of 1963 (WHO, 1963b). It was recognized that neither clinical practice nor medical education based on former principles of clinical medicine could create the physician of tomorrow; and that more consideration needed to be given to man as a person and as a member of a larger group, whose health and sickness were intimately connected with the conditions of life in the home and at work.

In one or two countries, notably India and Mexico, special orientation courses based on village studies and on the epidemiology of diseases in particular rural areas have prepared professional health personnel to recognize and work within an unfamiliar set of conditions. Orientation to local cultural and environmental influences on health and on prevalent attitudes to new health programmes also takes place at the international centres for medical research and training. There are, however, a number of potential opportunities that have yet to be recognized and used in order that the total health services of developing countries may achieve maximum efficacy. The kind of approach to their work considered desirable for physicians by the World Health Assembly is equally valid for all health workers. Orientation and training of this kind have to cover health personnel who are nationals as well as expatriates; those who have professional standing in the services, and those who form the very large group called 'auxiliary' health workers; and the faculty of all medical, nursing, and health training centres and their students.

TRAINING IN THE SOCIAL SCIENCES FOR PROFESSIONAL HEALTH WORKERS

Here and there experiments are taking place to discover in what ways and at what stages of training social science courses can be effectively introduced in the professional preparation of physicians and other health workers. In the seminar held in Bogotá in 1964 it was pointed out that anthropology taught in the pre-medical years can arouse interest in the young student. This early orientation disposes him to observe and become familiar with the health problems and outlook of people whose cultural patterns and economic standards of living are very different from his own. On the other hand, when the insertion of social science courses is little more than lip-service to the idea that place should be given to them without conviction about their value, no useful purpose is served. In many countries there are few if any social scientists interested in relating their teaching to health problems and the preparation of health personnel.

It has been found that anthropological or other social science teaching can be most effective in postgraduate and refresher courses. At this stage the health worker is likely to be aware of the magnitude, variety, and intricacy of health problems in tropical rural areas. In the second place, he will be only too conscious of the fact that his advice and teaching often fall on deaf ears, and few, if any, positive lasting results can be seen from his work. Finally, he may be aware that there ought to be a key to understanding the attitudes of rural people towards their health problems – if only he could find it.

It is likely, therefore, that social science courses adapted to the health needs of the area will provide him with clues to some of the problems he already recognizes. They may also indicate problems of which he is only half aware. It is important that such courses should give all participants ample time and opportunity to state, examine, analyse, and reflect on the local health problems encountered in their work. This aspect needs to be carefully considered at the planning stage; if it is well carried out it can be the most educative part of the course. Associated with this technique of problem analysis is the use of case studies by the professor in his teaching. They may form sources of reading material for the students, as well as indicate how they might organize the presentation of their own field problems. One of the main difficulties in these courses is to throw the net wide enough to include a number of aspects of rural living, which students may not at first recognize as having relevance to health problems. Although part of the value of the courses lies in the students' own analysis of local problems as they have seen them, a course would fail in its purpose unless it opened up new angles on the lives of rural people and communities. Some reports on the progress of community development projects and their evaluation could be used in this connexion.

SPECIAL PROBLEMS IN
TRAINING AUXILIARY HEALTH WORKERS

The problems in orientation faced by the faculty in training centres for auxiliary workers were discussed in the WHO conference on the training of health auxiliary personnel in Khartoum in 1961. It was emphasized that auxiliary health workers are the last link, but often the most important, in the chain between the health service and the people, and their training should be designed to help them to bridge the gulf that often exists between the scientific concepts of public health and the folklore of the people. An understanding of the people among whom the auxiliary will work should be one of the main elements in his training, and he should be given help and practice in relating the technical material of his course to the actual life and habits of the community. The auxiliary is often in a unique position to study the level of health consciousness of the people in his community and to discover, in the course of conversations during his daily work, what are regarded as serious health problems.

A warning needs to be given about the widely held idea that local personnel, trained and employed in their own area, will know all about the communities that they serve. Such individuals may be aware of certain practices relating to health situations, but they do not as a rule know in any systematic way about the social organization of their own people, nor about their cultural patterns of living. Moreover, as a result of scientific health training, they are sometimes ashamed of admitting that certain local practices exist and may try to conceal them. They may be still more reluctant to admit any knowledge of why people follow such practices, except to ascribe it to the 'superstition of the uneducated peasants'.

THE NEED FOR LIAISON WITH FIELD RESEARCH

No effective orientation and training courses in the application of social science concepts and techniques can be planned without the use of and constant reference to current field research. This research may be in the hands of individual social science research workers; it may be conducted under the guidance of local or foreign university departments; or it may be channelled through a local social science research institute. There are very few countries as yet where any effective liaison exists between on-going research in non-medical fields and the preparation of health workers. This lack of liaison is only too obvious in the content of some of the curricula for the teaching of social science in public health training courses. The kind of research material needed has been indicated in Part II of this book. Its application to public health work necessitates also detailed local knowledge about such conditions as food habits, birth practices and child-rearing, folk medicine and its uses, the skills used by traditional practitioners, and so on. Furthermore, it includes the relation of this body of knowledge about health practices and health conditions to general agricultural and economic conditions; and both the health and the general living conditions have to be related to the process and speed of social and cultural change. The speed of change can render some aspects of research in cultural fields out of date, as is seen in the changing attitudes towards curative services and the use of hospitals in some areas. Change, however, is often uneven in its impact on people's response, as many illustrations in this book have shown. The lesson to be learned here by health personnel and by social scientists is that all new health plans must be tuned to changing conditions, and that the nature and process of these changes demand constant vigilance.

References

References

ABDOU, S. & OMRAN, A. R. (n.d.) Some health education aspects of bilhar-ziasis control in Egypt. (Unpublished paper.)

ADAIR, J. (1958). The process of innovation and the Navaho–Cornell Field Health Research Project. Paper to Social Science Research Council committee on preventive medicine and social science research. June. (Unpublished.)

ADAIR, J. (1963). Physicians, medicine men and their Navaho patients. In Iago Galdston (ed.), *Man's image in medicine and anthropology*. New York: International Universities Press.

ADAIR, J., DEUSCHLE, K. & MCDERMOTT, W. (1957). Patterns of health and disease among the Navahos. *Ann. Amer. Acad. polit. soc. Sci.* **311**, 86.

ADAMS, R. N. (1963). Changing dietary and health practices. Paper to UN Conference on Science and Technology, Geneva. February. (Mimeo.)

AMMAR, H. (1954). *Growing up in an Egyptian village*. London: Rout-ledge & Kegan Paul.

AMMAR, H. (1960). The sociological approach to problems of community development. Arab States Fundamental Education Centre, Sirs-el-Layyan, U.A.R.

ATTIAH, M. A. H., EL KHOLY, A. & OMRAN, A. H. (1962). Beliefs and atti-tudes regarding communicable eye diseases and their control procedures in a rural community. *Bull. Ophthalmic Soc. of Egypt* **55**, 1–15.

BABIKER, K. & BESHIR EL SHEIKH (1962). An evaluation of health programmes in the Gezira irrigated area. Ministry of Health, Sudan.

BANERJI, D. & ANDERSON, S. (1962). Awareness of symptoms among cases of pulmonary tuberculosis in a district in South India. National Tuberculosis Institute, India.

BHARARA, S. S. (1961). Public attitudes in relation to small pox eradica-tion. Health Education Bureau, Lucknow, U.P.

BHARARA, S. S. (1962). Pilot health education and reorientation training. Health Education Bureau, Lucknow, U.P.

BROTMACHER, L. (1955). Medical practice among the Somali. *Bull. Hist. Med.* **29**, 197–229.

BROWN, M. S. (1957). Report of training course in health education. South Pacific Commission, Noumea.

References

BURGESS, A. (1960). Nutrition education in public health programmes: What have we learned? *Amer. J. publ. Hlth.* **51**, 1715–26.

BURGESS, A. & DEAN, R. F. A. (eds.) (1962). *Malnutrition and food habits.* London: Tavistock Publications; New York: Macmillan.

BURTON, J. (1961). Health education and the culture of communities. In W. Hobson (ed.), *Theory and practice of public health.* London: Oxford University Press. Pp. 336–42.

CARSTAIRS, G. M. (1955). Medicine and faith in rural Rajasthan. In B. D. Paul (ed.), *Health, culture and community.* Russell Sage Foundation.

CARSTAIRS, G. M. (1957). *The twice born.* London: Hogarth.

CLARK, M. (1959). *Health in the Mexican American culture.* Berkeley, Calif.: University of California Press.

DEPARTMENT OF HEALTH AND WELFARE, STATE OF ALASKA (1962). The McGrath Project. Report of a demonstration study on the prevention of upper respiratory diseases.

DE SANDOVAL, G. H. (1963). Study to determine the type of obstetrical care given to the population of sanitary sub-district IX in Mexico D.F. (Unpublished English typescript.)

DEUSCHLE, K. (1963). Training and use of medical auxiliaries in a primitive rural community. Paper to UN Conference on Science and Technology, Geneva. February. (Mimeo.)

DHILLON, H. S. & KARM, S. B. (1961). Investigation of cultural patterns and beliefs among tribal populations in Orissa with regard to malaria eradication activities. Central Health Education Bureau, New Delhi.

DUBE, S. C. (1955). *Indian village.* Routledge & Kegan Paul.

EAST AFRICAN INSTITUTE OF SOCIAL RESEARCH (1959). Symposium at Makerere University College, Kampala, Uganda. (Mimeographed papers.)

ERASMUS, C. J. (1961). *Man takes control.* Minneapolis: University of Minnesota Press.

FIELD, M. J. (1960). *Search for security.* London: Faber.

FOSTER, G. M. (1958). Problems in intercultural health programmes. Pamphlet No. 12, Social Science Research Council. New York.

GADALLAH, F. R. A. (1962). Some cultural implications in medical and public health practice in Egypt. *J. Egypt. Publ. Hlth. Assoc.* **37**, No. 3.

GANEWATTE, P. (1962). Health education project in Batagama rural community, Ceylon. Paper to research symposium at International Conference on Health and Health Education, Philadelphia. July. See Vol. 5, pp. 618–21, of report published by *Internat. J. Hlth. Educ.*, 1963.

GÉBER, M. & DEAN, R. F. A. (1956). The psychological changes accompanying kwashiorkor. *Courrier* **4**, No. 1.

References

GELFAND, M. & WILD, H. (1955). The Nyanga of Mashonaland. *Central African J. Med.* **1**, Nos. 3, 4, 5, 6.

GELFAND, M. & WILD, H. (1959). Some native herbal remedies in use in Mashonaland. *Central African J. Med.* **5**.

GERLACH, L. P. (1961). Economy and protein malnutrition among the Digo. *Proc. Minnesota Acad. Sci.* **29**, 3–13.

GERLACH, L. P. (1963). Traders on bicycles. *Sociologus* **13**, No. 1. (Berlin.)

GOULD, H. A. (1957). The implications of technical change for folk and scientific medicine. *Amer. Anthrop.* **50**, 507.

GROEN, J. J., BEN-ISHAY, D. & BEN-ASSA, B. I. (1962). Clinical and biochemical osteomalacia among the Bedouin of the Negev Desert. *Voeding* **23**, 49–61.

HARVEY, T. E. C. & ARMITAGE, F. B. (1961). Some herbal remedies and observations on the Nyanga of Matabeleland. *Central African J. Med.* **7**, No. 6.

JELLIFFE, D. B. (1957). Cultural blocks and protein malnutrition in early childhood in West Bengal. *Pediatrics* **20**, July.

JELLIFFE, D. B. & BENNETT, F. J. (1960). Indigenous medical systems and child health. *J. Pediatrics* **57**, 248–58.

KARUNARATNE, A. W. & GANEWATTE, P. (1964). Community participation in housing and environmental hygiene in Ceylon. In *Housing programmes: the role of public health agencies.* WHO Public Health Papers No. 25.

KELLY, I. (1954). The Bienstar social rural programme. (Mimeo.)

KELLY, I. (1960). An approach to the improvement of diet. Background paper for conference on Malnutrition and Food Habits, Cuernavaca, Mexico. For a report of the conference, see A. Burgess & R. F. A. Dean (eds.), *Malnutrition and food habits.* London: Tavistock Publications; New York: Macmillan, 1962.

KHARE, R. S. (1963). Folk medicine in a North Indian village. *Hum. Org.* **22**, No. 1.

LAMBO, T. A. (1963). African traditional beliefs, concepts of health and medical practice. Ibadan, Nigeria: Ibadan University Press.

LANTIS, M. L. (1957). American Arctic populations: their survival problem. In *Arctic Biology*, 18th Biology Colloquium held at Oregon State College. Pp. 119–30.

LANTIS, M. L. (1959). Folk medicine and hygiene in the Lower Kuskokwim and Nunivak Nelson Islands areas. *Anthrop. papers Univ. Alaska* **8**, No. 1, December.

LANTIS, M. L. (1962). Alaska village sanitation programme at the end of five years. Arctic Health Research Centre, Anchorage, Alaska.

References

LEIGHTON, A. H. & LAMBO, T. A. (1963). Psychiatric problems in developing countries. Paper to UN Conference on Science and Technology, Geneva. February. (Mimeo.)

LOISON, G. (1960). Pour une politique concrète d'éducation sanitaire en Afrique Equatoriale. *Rev. Hyg. Méd. soc.* **8**, No. 3. (Paris.)

LOUDON, J. B. (1957). Social structure and health concepts among the Zulu. *Hlth. Educ. J.* **15**, 90–98.

LYONS, F. MAXWELL (1960). Trachoma. *Practitioner* **185**, 33–40.

MCDERMOTT, W., DEUSCHLE, K., ADAIR, J., FULMER, H. & LOUGHLIN, B. (1960). Introducing modern medicine in a Navaho community. *Science* **131**, Nos. 3395 and 3396.

MARKOVIĆ, B. (1962). Typhoid gives way to education. Paper to International Conference on Health and Education, Philadelphia. July. See Vol. 3, pp. 363–8, of report published by *Internat. J. Hlth. Educ.*, 1963.

MESSENGER, J. C. (1959). Religious acculturation among the Anang-Ibibio. In W. Bascom and M. J. Herskovits (eds.), *Continuity and change in African cultures*. Chicago: University of Chicago Press.

MIYASAKA, T. (1962). An evaluation of a demonstration project in public health in a rural area in Japan. Paper to research symposium at International Conference on Health and Health Education, Philadelphia. July. See Vol. 5, pp. 631–4, of report published by *Internat. J. Hlth. Educ.*, 1963.

OPLER, M. E. (1963). The cultural definition of illness in village India. *Hum. Org.* **22**, 32–5.

OTTENBERG, P. (1959). Changing economic position of women among the Afikpo Ibo. In W. Bascom and M. J. Herskovits (eds.), *Continuity and change in African cultures*. Chicago: University of Chicago Press.

PAUL, B. D. (ed.) (1955). *Health, culture and community*. Russell Sage Foundation.

PEARSALL, M. (1962). Some behavioral factors in the control of TB in a rural county. *Amer. Rev. Respiratory Dis.* **84**, No. 2.

PRICE-WILLIAMS, D. R. (1962). The changing ideas of health and disease among the Tiv of Central Nigeria. Paper to research symposium at International Conference on Health and Health Education, Philadelphia. July. See Vol. 5, pp. 554–7, of report published by *Internat. J. Hlth. Educ.*, 1963.

PRINCE, R. (1961). Some notes on Yoruba native doctors and their management of mental illness. Paper for the First Pan-African Psychiatric Conference, Aro, Nigeria.

READ, M. (1956). *The Ngoni of Nyasaland*. London: Oxford University Press.

References

READ, M. (1957). Social and cultural backgrounds for planning public health programmes in Africa. WHO Regional Office for Africa, Brazzaville.

READ, M. (1959). Home, school and community in health education activities. Background paper for joint WHO/UNESCO Expert Committee on Teacher Preparation for Health Education. November. (Unpublished.)

READ, M. (1960). *Children of their fathers: growing up among the Ngoni.* New Haven, Conn.: Yale University Press.

READ, M. (1962). Man in his social environment. Paper to International Conference on Health and Health Education, Philadelphia. July. See Vol. 4, pp. 383–93, of report published by *Internat. J. Hlth. Educ.,* 1963.

SABER, M. (1962). Cultural change and community development. (English introduction to Arabic book.) Arab States Fundamental Education Centre, Sirs-el-Layyan, U.A.R.

SAUNDERS, L. (1962). The contributions and limitations of behavioral sciences in public health. In *The behavioral sciences and public health.* Continuing Education Monographs, No. 3, Western Regional Office, American Public Health Association, San Francisco.

SCUDDER, T. (1962). *The ecology of the Gwembe Tonga.* Kariba Studies, Vol. 2. Manchester: Manchester University Press.

SHARMA, D. C. (1955). Mother, child and nutrition. *J. trop. Pediatrics* 1, June.

SIMMONS, O. G. (1955). Popular and modern medicine in Mestizo communities of coastal Peru and Chile. *J. Amer. Folklore* 68, 57.

SOLIEN, N. L. & SCRIMSHAW, H. S. (1957). Public health significance of child feeding practices observed in a Guatemalan village. *J. trop. Pediatrics* 3, 99.

SOMESWARA RAO, K., SWAMINATHAN, M. C., SWARUP, S. & PATWARDHAN, V. N. (1959). (Nutrition Research Laboratories, Indian Council of Medical Research, Coonoor, South India.) Protein malnutrition in South India. *Bull. Wld. Hlth. Org.* 20, 603–39.

SPENS, T. (1960). Social aspects of a health education programme in Trans-Volta Togoland. Paper to seminar on Social and Technological Change, Institute of Commonwealth Studies, London. (Unpublished.)

SPILLIUS, J. (1962). Environmental sanitation in Tonga. Paper to research symposium at International Conference on Health and Health Education, Philadelphia. July. See Vol. 5, pp. 560–3, of report published by *Internat. J. Hlth. Educ.,* 1963.

TANNER, R. E. S. (1959). Sukuma leechcraft. *East African med. J.* 36, February.

TENTORI, F. V. (1962). Their needs and knowledge. *Internat. J. Hlth. Educ.* 5.

References

WADDY, B. B. (1962). The present state of public health in the African Soudan. *Transact. Roy. Soc. trop. Med. Hyg.* **56**, 95–115.

WELLIN, E. (1953). Pregnancy, childbirth and midwifery in the valley of Ica, Peru. Memorandum prepared by Ica Anthropology Project. June. (Unpublished.)

WHO (1953). First International Symposium on yaws control. WHO Monograph Series No. XV.

WHO (1958). Medical rehabilitation. First report of Expert Committee. WHO Technical Reports Series No. 158.

WHO (1963a). *WHO Chronicle* **17**, No. 8, 305–8.

WHO (1963b). Preventive medicine and the physician. *WHO Chronicle* **17**, No. 9, 350–8.

WILSON, M. (1957). *Rituals of kinship among the Nyakyusa.* London: Oxford University Press.

WISER, C. (1963). *Behind mud walls 1930–1960.* Berkeley, Calif.: University of California Press.

ZELLEKE, S. M. (1962). Fighting the 'king of diseases'. Paper to International Conference on Heath and Health Education, Philadelphia. July. See Vol. 2, pp. 162–7, of report published by *Internat. J. Hlth. Educ.*, 1963.

Index

Index